For the Asking

a joyful journey to peace

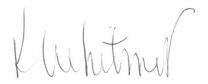

Also by Kathleen Whitmer

Green Rubber Boots:
A Joyful Journey to Wellness

What readers say about *For the Asking*

"A story of hope, healing and peace."

– Mary Mounta, Ft, Myers, Florida

———————————

"*For the Asking…* is in every way splendid…personal,
honest, and energized."

– Father Eugene Linehan,
Georgetown Preparatory School, N. Bethesda, Maryland

———————————

"Thank you for caring so much about a perfect stranger
who had lost her way."

– Joan Mottice, Akron, Ohio

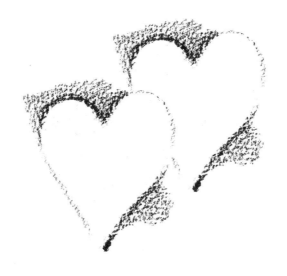

Each heart knows its own joy.

On the cover

Moonlight Magic
oil on linen, 60″ x 60″ by Kathleen Whitmer

Editors

Rose A.O. Kleidon
Kurt Kleidon

Book design

The cover design and interior layout design for
For the Asking: A Joyful Journey to Peace are
by Christie Lang.

Type design

This book is typeset in Adobe Caslon, designed by Carol
Twombly. It is a revival of a typeface designed and cut by
William Caslon in England in the 18th Century.

For the Asking

a joyful journey to peace

Written and illustrated by

Kathleen Whitmer

Foreword by Bob Dyer, *Omar! My Life On and Off the Field*

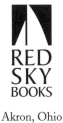

RED
SKY
BOOKS

Akron, Ohio

For the Asking

a joyful journey to peace

Author's Note: While the stories are about real people, their names have been changed.

Books may be purchased in quantity for educational, business or sales promotion use. Please write Special Promotions, Kleidon Publishing, 320 Springside Drive, Akron, Ohio 44333.

SECOND PRINTING

ISBN 0–9661079–4–2 (Limited Edition, hard bound)
ISBN 0-9712941-2-7 (pbk.)

Library of Congress Cataloging-in-Publication Data:
   Whitmer, Kathleen.
   For the asking: a joyful journey to peace/
   Kathleen Whitmer. — 1st ed.
   p. cm.

   1. Spiritual biography. 2. Prayer. 3. Organ Transplant. 4. Whitmer, Kathleen. 5. Wellness. 6. Happiness.

Library of Congress Control Number: 2002105552

PRINTED IN THE UNITED STATES OF AMERICA

Dedication

With much love and gratitude, I wish to
dedicate this book to my husband, Jerry.
He never lost faith in me. He traveled the
journey to peace every step of the way,
and

I thank my sister and my good friends,
Mary Ann Bamberger,
Donamari Guy,
Alberta Schumacher,
Kay Riley,
and
Jean Tremelin
and

the kind words of encouragement from:
Eugene Linehan, S.J.,
Cecilia Nagel, C.S.J.
and

finally the donor of my new heart
and

Randall Starling, M.D.,
and all the doctors and staff of
The Cleveland Clinic Foundation.

Contents

Contents

Poems

"May the God of hope
fill you with joy and peace
in believing that you
may abound in hope by the
power of the Holy Spirit."

Romans 15:13

Foreword

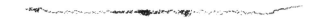

by Bob Dyer
Reprinted with permission of the *Akron Beacon Journal*

Kathleen "Boo" Whitmer is gazing out a window on the ninth floor of the Cleveland Clinic. It is a gorgeous morning in late May, sunny and warm and crystal-clear, the kind of day when you're thrilled just to be alive. Whitmer is barely alive. Her heart – battered by experimental cancer therapy decades earlier – has stopped producing oxygen. She is hooked to a needle that is pumping her with a special drug. She feels OK, considering she has been wired up since May 26. But she isn't going anywhere until somebody else stops living. "It's the weirdest thing to look outside and know you're not going to be out there again without somebody else's heart," she says.

The talented Akron artist and writer is one of 62,000 Americans desperately clinging to life while waiting for an organ. She's not the type of person to "root" for fatal accidents. Instead, she reminds herself that some things just can't be controlled. That enables her to retain the inner calm that has seen her through so many other medical traumas.

Whitmer has been on the waiting list for two years. Her condition has steadily deteriorated, and by May her test numbers were so bad she was immediately hospitalized.

Now fast-forward to the middle of June 1999.

Whitmer's long wait has ended. She has just returned to the airy, contemporary ranch near Portage Country Club in West Akron – with a new heart beating inside her.

Her cheeks are pink again. Some of the wrinkles seem to have disappeared. Soon, the perpetual exhaustion she felt with her old heart will be gone, too.

Whitmer has no clue where the new heart came from. She may never know. But now she has an affirmative answer to her most pressing question: Would she receive a heart before her clock ran out?

"The unknown is a real big part of all of this," she says softly. "And we don't like the unknown. We think we want to be in control. But once you relax and let the unknown take care of itself, it's just amazing how it does."

"Along with all of this journey comes a wonderful peace."

People like Kathleen Whitmer are the reason my driver's license contains a "organ donor" stamp. If I am decapitated tomorrow by a meteorite, I want the doctors to yank out any salvageable organs and stick them into people who need them. Why should I hang on to my organs when I'm dead?

If you think the same way, you need to make your wishes known. Putting the "organ donor" symbol on your license might not be enough. Most doctors tread with caution unless a family member gives approval, and speed is absolutely critical. So tell your family now.

"These things really do go on, and they're successful," says Whitmer, formerly an art teacher at Akron's Simon Perkins Junior High, a professor in the School of Art at Kent State University and an artist-in-residence at Old Trail School. "It's not something prehistoric or ghoulish. It's a matter of fact."

Heart transplants have become almost matter-of-fact at the Cleveland Clinic, which has performed over 800 since 1984. Across the country, 83 percent of the heart recipients now survive the first year.

Donors and recipients must match up not only in blood type, but in size. "I've got a little heart," says Whitmer.

Baloney. At least 5,000 book buyers know that's not the case. Whitmer has a huge heart, as is evident in the pages of *Green Rubber Boots: A Joyful Journey to Wellness,* the surprisingly uplifting story of her days as a human guinea pig.

In 1979, Whitmer was diagnosed with a rare form of sarcoma cancer and shipped off to the National Cancer Institute's research program in Bethesda, Md. After two surgeries, eight weeks of radiation and megadoses of experimental chemotherapy, she was still ticking – and by 1985 was declared completely cancer-free. But the drugs trashed her ticker.

If you know Whitmer, you already know she wants to make contact with the donor's family. But that procedure is delicate.

The flow of organs is controlled by a group called LifeBanc. LifeBanc offers the recipient a chance to write an anonymous thank-you letter. If the letter is up to snuff, the group forwards it. Names are exchanged only after that, and only if both sides are willing.

Even more dicey is the process of getting permission to harvest an organ in the immediate aftermath of an accident, when the victim's family is often overwhelmed with grief.

"It has to be done very, very carefully," Whitmer points out. "There are people who never would do it in a million years. Or maybe nobody's ever brought it up before."

The donation of a heart "is such a big gift," says one who knows. "And it's really kind of silly when you think about just putting it in the ground."

She's absolutely right. "Pass it on."

JUNE 27, 1999   BOB DYER
AKRON, OHIO

Bob Dyer is the author of Omar! My Life On and Off the Field. *This foreword appeared originally in the* Akron Beacon Journal.

Preface

For years I have carried with me the idea for this book. Since I completed my first book, *Green Rubber Boots: A Joyful Journey to Wellness*, three years ago, I have continued to write. I find myself with a deep yearning and need to organize my thoughts and watch them unfold.

Writing this book has become a blessing, a true gift from God. The inspiration and support for this book came from being ill and from being with the ill. We cannot force an idea or the desire on ourselves, we must be part of it. It does not come from the outside. It comes from within.

Finding peace within ourselves is a lifetime of work. Wanting to pray, learning to pray, feeling sad about always leaving it last in our day are a part of all of us. There are times in my life when I wanted to know what to say; my relationship with God was dry, cold, shallow. I longed to have God and his son, Jesus Christ, as my friends. I so wanted to feel their presence. I wanted to love them deeply. I wanted to follow them closely. Yet, I was always removed, busy.

My cancer experience took me to Naples, Florida, to help with my recovery in the early eighties. I can vividly remember a bright, sunny day sitting alone in a quiet, peaceful church. I sat still. I wanted something to happen. I longed to love more deeply, to be open to goodness, to make peace and love a way of life. How could I clear my head to make room for my God and all He is? I felt hopeless that day. I was alone in the church and alone inside myself.

The overwhelming loneliness of that day haunts me. I was empty. Illness and tough times awoke me from the sleep of a prayerless life. I had to ask God to help me make room for Him in what had been what I realize today a lifetime of struggling with prayer. I had to stop re-saying the same things. I had to stop in my tracks and listen. He came to me ever so gently with the words and the way to Him.

The thunder, the lightning, the storms of our lives bring with them silence. In that silence of sickness, I found how to pray. When we are ill, we do, indeed, pray differently. As I write this introduction, this book has already been written. Strange, one would think an introduction would come first in the process. However, for me, it has been the opposite. What I might have written at the start of this rewarding task is very different today. I knew not where my yellow pencil would take me.

Written prayer is powerful. Prayer written in pain is truth. Prayer in progress is never-ending. Prayer life is like all of life. It grows; it changes; it deepens. With practice it becomes better and better, no longer a burden, but a joy. No longer put at the end of a long day but included throughout the morning, the afternoon, and the evening into night.

Welcome to *For the Asking: A Joyful Journey to Peace*. It has been designed and written in order that your journey to becoming healthier in all aspects of your life will be comforting and consoling.

Illness gives us that surplus of time when we can look back in peace and quiet and reflect on the events of our lives. Reflections, short stories, thoughts, along with prayers and quotations are scattered at random throughout this book in order that you may use them to help you relax, ponder, be well, or just simply smile.

Believe and welcome amusing things stored in all our memories that return in vivid detail just when we need them the most. They help to lighten the load of pain, loneliness and discomfort.

Included are short stories which were written and published in a local newspaper, *Focus on Mature Lifestyles*. They have no chronological order, nor do they have any relationship with each other. They simply reflect the kinds of things we remember, the experiences we share. They are stories of life. Quite simply, they are the celebration of life in the present.

I was encouraged to include them because they bring happiness and laughter and a new voice to the lines of print.

"Dress Rehearsal" tells of an anxious, middle-of-the-night venture to receive a new heart. It moves us into a world about which we have wondered.

"Blue Ribbon Cat," written in the voice of a cat, tells the humorous story of shopping for a new cat. Eloquently spoken, the cat tells of his own joys of life. The break from my own voice is intended to bring realization to the treasures of everyday gifts.

"Color Your World Happy" is intended to heighten things learned but sometimes forgotten. Life cannot move us from our internal joy unless we permit it!

"Tommy's Angel" is a delightful memory of Tom and his calorie-impaired guardian angel. The memories that are part of our lives enrich today.

"So Much to Say" reflects on the observation of aging people and how they communicate. They remind us to say the things of today.

"Change My Range" tells of the way husbands and wives look at the same things in very different ways. Valuing the ways of others in our lives can give us direction and joy.

"And Then She Flew Out the Window" tells of an unbelievable story of a most precocious sibling. You will enjoy the outcome.

The thoughts in this book vary in length from long to just one line. They are meant to greet you where you are.

They are intended to make prayer real. They speak to our God in earnest requests and appreciation. They address divinity. They are calm, quiet and devoid of strife. They are intended to preserve in your heart a place where dreams and hopes can grow. The heart of prayer is what makes the world spin.

In days of illness or stress or pain, we are able to pray but a few words. Other days carry with them a need for much more.

You, my readers, mean much to me. I had not realized the "you" I have come to know since the publication of *Green Rubber Boots: A Joyful Journey to Wellness.* Phone messages at midnight from Milwaukee or Chicago humble me. The mailman brings messages, some long and detailed, others almost abbreviated. Yet, all from people like you. It startles me how small my world has become.

Six months after the publication of *Green Rubber Boots: A Joyful Journey to Wellness,* I wandered by a lady sitting on the beach in Florida. She was beautifully bronzed. She was the picture of health and relaxation. She was seated not more than ten feet from the spot where I began to write *Green Rubber Boots* two years earlier.

As I looked closely, I saw that she was reading my book. It was tattered and worn. It had seen better days. I laughed because I never get to see my books once they have been read and passed along.

That simple experience was, for me, God's way of affirming that He was part of my writing. I was doing His work. He was speaking to me – I had listened. He encouraged me to continue to speak through the written word. His words travel from my fingers through my yellow pencil onto my yellow legal pad. I am but His messenger.

♡ *The prayer of the monk is not perfect until he no longer recognizes himself or the fact that he is praying.*

St. Anthony

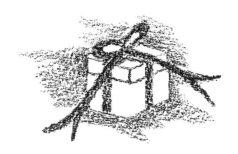

Across the Hall

I wish I could have helped the lady across the hall from my ninth floor hospital room. One morning when five or six doctors left her room, she pulled the drapes and closed the door to her room. All day hospital personnel rapped gently on her door before entering. They tiptoed in quietly with her medicines and food.

She had received bad news. There was nothing more they could do for her. Her heart had completely deteriorated. It could not be repaired. Her body would not tolerate a heart transplant. She had reached the end of the medical maze. The doctors were gentle, kind, and apologetic.

All day I watched. I worried. I wondered. My nurse was her nurse. As evening descended, the room darkened. A dull gray consumed her room. Her dinner tray was removed untouched. She was to go home in the morning.

This, one of the finest cardiac hospitals in the nation, could not help her. She had so much she wanted to do. She wanted to enjoy her grandchildren. She wanted to laugh and sing. She wanted to work in her garden. What was it like for her to hear the words of the heart doctors? Hope was no more. What is life like with no hope?

Morning broke. Her drapes parted. Her breakfast tray was received. She waved a little greeting to me as she peeked from her hospital room. The day of quiet and darkness, alone with You, had helped her to accept the bleak future.

By mid-afternoon her family arrived. She was to go home and live out her final days saying her good-byes. It was easy to see that You had spent that last day in the hospital with her. You prepared her. She was able to accept what was to be. Will You give me that same strength when I need it?

She smiled as she left her room. Our eyes met for just one brief moment. We knew we would see one another again. Her love for You shone all around her. From her fragile body radiated the assurance that You would care for her. The days ahead would be kind. Her courage helped me greatly. When my days are numbered, please give me the same gift of acceptance that You gave the lady across the hall.

♡ *In your books were written all the days that were formed for me, when none of them yet existed.*

Psalm 139:16

God Knows Best

Today I realize that as a child I prayed as a child. In fact, I can clearly remember being taught that there are two kinds of prayer: prayers of petition and prayers of thanksgiving. And so, when Grandma Casey was sick, we asked God to make her well. Our childhood prayers were full of asking for things, for favors, for wellness. Then the prayers of thanksgiving followed those prayers. Sometimes our prayers of petition weren't answered in a positive way, but we said thank you, no matter what, because God knew best, and He would do what He knew He had planned, and we were to say thank you for just the listening part.

Childhood prayer and adolescent prayer were about the same. Someplace along the way I decided to just stop that

Ping-Pong® kind of prayer life, and I started saying, "Thy will be done." Just when that all started, I am not sure.

Perhaps we grow in spirituality just as we do physically. Many years ago I grew tired of my prayer books. They became boring and repetitious. My prayer life was that of a child. I was still asking for guidance, health, things to turn out just fine, and still following with prayers of thanksgiving.

It was not until I had spent months seriously ill, in a small hospital room at the Cleveland Clinic that I realized how out of touch my prayers were. On one early May morning as I awoke and looked out the window of my cozy ninth floor room at the view of downtown Cleveland that I had grown to like, I realized that my spiritual growth had taken on new meaning. The wait for a new heart had its benefits. In the silence of my new life style, I was more in tune with God than ever before in my life. By leaps and bounds my prayers took on new form. I had grown up. God heard me as the adult I am.

He, too, had gotten a little bored and tired of prayers of petition and thanksgiving. He wanted me to be His friend. He wanted to talk with me. The glorious time had come when we were to have conversations. He had ever so gently placed me in my little room on the cardiac care floor of my new home. The Cleveland Clinic was to be our meeting place. The reasons for things became clear and bright. People asked how I could stand being cooped up and alone while waiting for a heart. It was easy. I was never alone. I was not bored or anxious. It was during this time that I recognized the major changes going on in my prayer life. My new prayer life led me in a different direction, one that gave form and substance to my hopefulness.

My new prayer life had nothing to do with what I prayed for. It is hard to put into words because it was no longer an activity but a state of being. It is more like a place I seek, in my mind, in my spirit: a place I go for peace with God, myself and the world.

As we walk our spiritual journey, we grasp for something we feel inside ourselves. As with all kinds of growth, there is difficulty. There are periods when we become stymied. Days, months, sometimes years go by as we stumble. Turmoil bears down on us. We move two steps backwards after moving three steps forward. We falter; we become complacent. My faith returned after a dry spell and presented itself as big as you please: bigger and stronger as though it had been in some physical fitness program.

Today when I awoke, dear Jesus, my room was filled with You. You waited patiently as rest nourished my tired body. I could feel the fullness of the room. Behind my closed eyes I whispered, "Good morning."

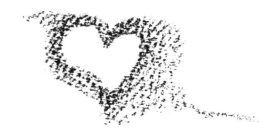

I Row and Row

When the rain came into my life,
  You gave me an umbrella.

When the rain poured,
  You sent me a boat.

Today I row and row closer to You.

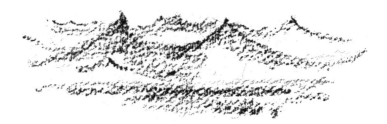

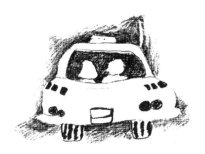

It's All Up To You

I am happiest when I am with You. With the days of running from one task to another, to the everyday outside world behind me, I now appreciate this short stay on Earth. In the peace and quiet of recovery, I feel more productive and more loving.

When my heart was damaged by the chemotherapy that was much too toxic for it to handle, it took me time to adjust to the new lifestyle it demanded. Slowing down was not easy. Denial sneaked into my thinking. The "maybe's" of being ill came easily. Maybe I will be better tomorrow. Maybe the doctor isn't quite right. I forged ahead. My heart grew big and swollen. At night, I could hear it working hard to keep my blood circulating. It labored in loud rhythm.

Gradually, the rhythm became uneven and unpredictable. I knew the truth. You gave me subtle clues that all was not well. You helped me listen to the unhealthy beats in the quiet of the night.

Anticipation of what would be ahead was heavy. A conversation with You helped to quiet my "what ifs" and "what will be's." As a set of stairs grew higher and a city block longer, I had to ask You for help. I was in trouble. I visited You more often. Your answers were clear. You gave me the gift of acceptance. The thumping in my chest became more labored. We talked about it. Clearly, You taught me about my body and the stress it was encountering. Ever so gradually, You led me through the medical maze. One step at a time, You directed me. You orchestrated the process. Moving from one doctor to another, one test to another, and one hospital to another was easy with You in the back seat of the car.

When a young cardiologist finally broke the news to my husband and me, You were there. When he announced that my own heart was ready to be replaced by a heart transplant, an awed moment of silence filled the room. Within seconds, I was able to say, "Let's get on with it." Where did I get the strength? From where had the courage come? You and I both know the answer. You had climbed out of the back seat of the car to accompany us to the appointment. You waited patiently. If You were able to be patient with all You have to do, certainly I could be patient too.

I was to get a new heart. Where were You going to find one? This is where I really turned it all over to You. This is where You moved into the driver's seat.

Thy Will Be Done

The sky is bright pink. From my ninth floor room in the Cleveland Clinic, I can see that the rooftops are covered with snow. I know not what tomorrow brings. Somehow yesterday's fear is gone. Your peace fills me. I pray this colorful evening that You have good things planned for tomorrow.

I am here to do Your will. Give me only the strength and the courage to endure whatever the outcome of the tests will be. Guide the hands of my surgeon. Bless those dedicated people who will ponder over my case and decide what is best. Be in on the plans, O Holy One. It is comforting to know that You are the director of this big task. I am excited to see what you have planned. "Thy will be done" fills my spirit. I long to feel Your touch.

The warmth of Your love is at the core of my body. I feel its comfort. Like the pink of tonight's sky, the beauty of the warmth of Your love fills me to the brim with the peace that You have given me. Thy will be done, O Lord. Thy will be done.

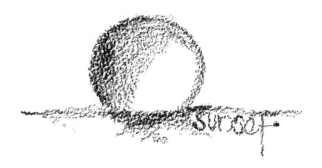

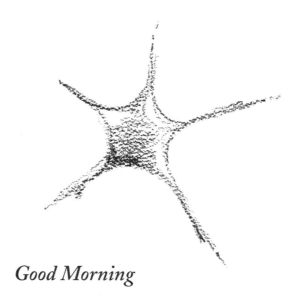

Good Morning

Good morning, dear God.
  The night sped by.
  You never left my side.
  In me You preside.

Good morning, dear God.
  Bless this day that is just beginning.
  Keep the world outside
  and the body in which I live at peace.

Good morning, dear God.
  I shall never fear,
  for you are near.
  You fill my day with Your light.

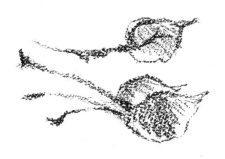

Color Your World Happy

We live in a society that worships youth and wellness. Perfect "abs" are a must. Are you as tired as I am of hearing about them? I haven't seen mine in years, and I haven't missed them.

Somewhere along the way, we seem to have come to the conclusion that youth plus wellness equals happiness. But is this necessarily true?

Today, turning forty brings with it black balloons, "over the hill" cards, and an array of wrinkle creams. Old is the enemy. Illness is dreaded.

The equation then is old plus ill equals unhappiness. More and more I become convinced how questionable this belief is.

Isn't it a misguided society that encourages panic at the thought of turning forty? We all know people can be young and healthy and miserable, and we can be old and not well and be joyfully happy.

Once we realize that happiness comes from the inside, to be nurtured and cared for, age and health become less important. We all know one miserable teenager and one delightfully joyful cancer patient.

Life is filled with the unknown and the not-so-good. But we cannot allow ourselves the luxury of saying, "Why me?" "Why not me?" makes more sense.

As I recently opened a new box of crayons, I was taken by how much people resemble crayons. We come into the world weighing within pounds of one another. We look alike and we are here for one ultimate purpose. We differ in small ways, yet, why do we spend much of our time dwelling on our differences?

Age and time alter the crayons. Some get broken, some stay sharp, some stay tall and straight, and some just wear out. But, all the crayons have a purpose: to make the world a more colorful, kinder place.

Like the crayons, some of us get tired or sick. Some of us stay whole. Yet our purpose remains: to take joy in God, one another and ourselves while making the world a good place.

Life is not simple, but how can make it less complicated?

♡ *I praise you for I am fearfully and wonderfully made. Wonderful are your works; that I know very well.*

Psalm 139:14

Heart to Heart

The printer of my books and I had a talk recently concerning prayer. We had a good laugh as we admitted how differently we pray when we are face to face with serious illness. All the kinds of prayers we did before being ill changed with the realization that bad things do happen to good people.

Our prayer life grows up; it gets very serious. I am sorry deep down inside that my prayer life was a bit on the shallow side as I sailed through my healthy life. You were always there. We spoke cordially every day. We were good friends. In those days I was aware of Your existence. We were polite and friendly. I loved You very much, and I was sure of Your love for me.

As my friend and I discussed the BIPD (before illness prayer days) and compared them to the AIPD (after illness prayer days), he slapped his knee and threw his head back in laughter and said, "Hey, God, we need to have a heart-to-heart talk!" Our once formal, quiet, polite talks became loud and clear conversation. Our ability to listen to Your replies became acute. We finally learned what real prayer is about! I am a bit ashamed that I was just formal and friendly in the BIPD.

Our heart-to-heart conversations of today are fulfilling, fun, real, and essential to my everyday life. I am sad that I missed the excitement of really knowing You years ago. Wellness can do that, I guess. Winging it alone seemed OK. The time I spent with You before sleep and on Sundays seemed enough. How wrong I was. How thankful I am for those AIPD.

The Hummingbird

This morning the hummingbird sat of the perch that is attached to its feeder. Her tiny body rested as she drank the sugary drink Jerry had prepared for her. Her red throat relaxed as she swallowed the nourishment. The white stripe around her small neck was clearly defined. What a beautiful creature she is! You put her outside our kitchen window, just for us to enjoy.

Memories of her visits over the years remind me that she never stopped moving her wings as she ate. She would nervously eat, all the time fluttering about, being careful to be able to quickly get away from harm. She had not learned to trust us.

How like the hummingbird we are! Oh, we can't hover

in the air as she can, nor can we fly at all! Like her, in our youthful, childlike ways, we once darted around from place to place – in, out, up, down. We were nervous and uncertain. We jumped from one flower to another. We looked around, not quite sure of much. We grew, we prayed, we had to learn to know You. We had to realize that it was OK to sit down and to relax. We had to learn to trust You. You would never let any harm come to us.

My morning with our hummingbird made me realize Your sincere goodness. That tiny, red-throated bird with the white ringed neck taught me much this morning.

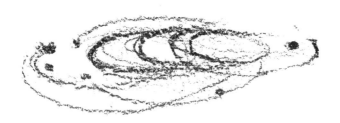

The Great Director

I rush through my early morning chores. I am eager to get to my writing. It has become apparent that the hours I spend writing this book are the hours I spend with You. It is prayer at its best. Verbal prayer is different from written prayer in that the thoughts are helter-skelter. In order to write prayer, I must plan, sort, and refine. How exciting it all is! It fascinates me how You work through us. You fill my mind with creativity. Mine is but to move the pencil as the ideas come from You. I have often prayed that I might spread Your word. You have shown me the way. You are the great Director. You lead us to You through one another.

Dress Rehearsal

The phone rang at 1:05 A.M. Why is the ring of the phone different when it shouts in the early morning, echoing in the darkness? There is a sense of fear and anxiety that accompanies its sound. Your brain shifts from peaceful dreams to stark reality with but a moment to switch gears. In the dark you reach for the spot making the familiar yet unfamiliar sound.

My hand found the receiver instantly. Knowing that I was on the heart transplant list at the Cleveland Clinic for seven months, I thought I was prepared for the call that would beckon me to Cleveland to receive a new heart!

Are we ever ready for the big things in our lives? Is knowing they are to happen ever enough?

In the dark that Sunday morning, the clear, sure voice on the line asked, "Is this Kathleen Whitmer?"

Even the voice of the questioner was what you would expect it should be. Strong, sure, it was the voice of a person in such a unique, important, life-saving position.

"Kathleen, we have found a heart for you. The procurement team has gone to Illinois to harvest it. We would like you to come to Cleveland Clinic as soon as you can."

– silence –

"Kathleen, are you awake?"

Kathleen wanted to say she wasn't Kathleen. "Kathleen ran away months ago. We can't find her," were replies that flashed through my mind for just one short moment.

"Yes, I am awake. Yes, I am Kathleen. Yes, I will be there. Would you like to speak with my husband for a moment?"

In the dark room, Jerry listened to the voice in authority. His responses were, "Yes, yes, yes, okay, yes, I understand."

– silence –

The dog and the cat were annoyed. They were settled in their favorite spots on the warm, downy comforter. Their graceful bodies moved as they seemed to know that this was not to be another warm, cozy night with the two people they loved the most.

For a short time, I turned into a four-year-old being told she had to eat octopus! "I don't know if I can do it! I don't know if I can do it," I haltingly spoke. Jerry, in his blue flannel pajamas, hugged me. His voice told me that he was as frightened as I was. His arms cradled me softly. We knew this day was coming, and now it was here.

My body started to shake. There was a lump in my throat. I needed to go to the bathroom. I had read about panic attacks; I had talked to people who had had them. This is what one was like. We turned on lights. We walked. We took deep breaths, and then without a hitch, realization set in. What I needed and what I wanted was about to happen! It was November 2, 1997. It was my lucky day!

Saturday, November 1, 1997, had been a restless day. I seemed not to be able to be still. Every little thing that needed to be done was done. Letters, notes, phone calls, groceries…the day was complete. Dinner was special. We had had a glass of wine together in our peaceful living room before dinner. We discussed our day. Jerry was energized by a legal seminar he had attended. I was excited by the return of my artwork from a month-long successful exhibition at a delightful local gallery.

After a call to my loving sister in New York, the preparation began. Since I had showered before going to bed, I calmly began by washing my hair and scrubbing my teeth. I put on my favorite, red, warm, fleece USA sweatshirt and a pair of my most comfortable blue jeans. I packed my toothbrush, favorite soap, slippers, and robe. Today's hospitals provide everything else.

By 1:30 A.M., I took one last glance at the home I loved. The dog and cat sat in the window together wondering where we were going. We never acted this way. Something special was happening. They seemed to know.

The streets of Cleveland were quiet. Our drive was easy. We were quiet. Now and then I would think of someone I wanted Jerry to call in the morning. I helped him memorize telephone numbers I had known for years. I made sure he knew that, if things did not go well, I loved him and I wanted him to be happy. Once we rounded the drive to the front door of the Cleveland Clinic, we were assured that not all of Cleveland was asleep. As we walked in, the guard at the door directed us to the Heart ICU Unit.

The walk was easy. I had turned it over to God. He would take care of me.

We entered the ICU unit through the automatic doors. Jerry said simply, "Kathleen Whitmer, heart transplant."

"Oh, the patient is not here yet," the nurse replied. "Let me make you comfortable while you await her arrival."

My mind raced. The patient is not here yet? "But I am the patient!" I said.

"You are?" asked the nurse. "Well, my name is Patty, over there is O.J., that is Mary Jane, and your nurse is going to be Oscar."

I had never before known a nurse named Oscar. The Oscar Mayer® hot dog jingle ran through my mind.

Then, with all the excitement and furor of people who do what they love to do, it was all set in motion. Oscar smiled. He was in heaven. O.J. proudly said, "It is, indeed, your lucky day!"

My bed was ready and waiting. On the crisp, white sheet lay the wires to the electrocardiogram. Suction cup circles were placed in the position where they were to be attached to my body. If I had had a magic marker with me, I could have played connect-the-dots and drawn a human figure on the bed.

Excitement, happiness. A wonderful, uplifting spirit filled the room. People who had had recent heart surgery lay in their beds, partially hidden behind clean white curtains that fell from metal tracks in the ceiling.

"They are preparing an operating room for you. One is being used right now. A patient is getting a new heart, lungs and a kidney. You'll be in the adjoining operating room. The team that went to Illinois for your heart will call before it starts back to Cleveland."

Someone in Illinois had died. That person died, and now with his or her heart, I would be able to live a normal, active life again. The bigness of it silenced me. At sixty-one years of age, I grew up never dreaming things such as this could or would ever happen. I thought of the people I knew who had gone before me. Somehow I felt their presence. They gave me strength. If all went wrong, they were there to greet me. I could feel their strength.

Teams of people in the middle of the night. The pilot, doctors and nurses, flying to Illinois for me. The "me" they did not even know. A crew of people preparing an operating room for heart transplant surgery for me. The "me" they didn't even know.

IV poles, monitors, all sorts of equipment surrounded my bed. Oscar gave me a hospital gown.

"Well, we can get started now," he said. We were getting started for the journey of my life.

I had had cancer and two long, grueling surgeries eighteen years earlier. I had had weeks of linear radiation, and I had had nine months of experimental chemotherapy (which had initially damaged my heart) at the National Institutes of Health. But nothing had prepared me for the moments that lay ahead.

I reached under my warm, red fleece USA sweatshirt, ready to release my left arm from its sleeve. A phone rang. Like toys with run-down batteries, everyone stopped.

– silence –

Oscar answered the little white phone that was attached to the side of my bed.

"Yes, yes, yes, okay, okay," we all heard him say. Suspense filled the room. "You can go home now. The heart in Illinois is not healthy. It has a clogged artery."

Shoulders slumped. The quiet was heavy. O.J. said, "Well, I guess it is your lucky day after all. You don't need an unhealthy heart. You already have one of those."

Oscar gave me a chair on which to sit. We all just looked from one to another. "The chief of transplant teams refused the heart," repeated Oscar as he held his fist tight indicating the clogged artery. "Clogged artery, no good."

We left the hospital by the same route we had entered. Driving down Euclid Avenue at 3:00 A.M. felt surrealistic.

We had not shopped or dined. We had gone for a new heart. We had gone through the process. I had put my toe in the water. We had had a dress rehearsal.

We drove back to Akron as quietly as we had driven to Cleveland. At 4:00 A.M., we climbed back into our bed. The dog and cat had warmed our spots. Tomorrow would be another day.

Life would not be the same. The experience was a once-in-a-lifetime experience. We had ridden a roller coaster. We were ready for the inevitable. We were energized by those good people who love the unknown. They are risk-takers. They are ready for the unpredictable. They take joy in living their lives so that others will someday be healthy.

Indeed, tomorrow will be another day. The phone will ring again. I am ready. God knows when it will be. I can relax. I am better prepared than I was before 1:05 A.M., Sunday, November 2, 1997.

♡ *Honor physicians for their services, for the Lord created them;*
for their gift of healing comes from the Most High.

Sirach 38:1–2

27

In the Morning

In the morning the new day arises.
  By noon it is in full bloom.
  By mid-afternoon it begins to be quiet.
  By dusk it softens.
  By night it goes to rest.

Darkness descends only to dawn again
  that we may take joy
  in the light of another day.

Thank You, Lord.

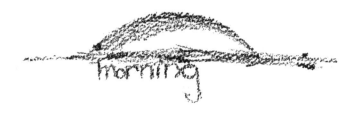

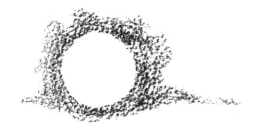

Free with the Truth

When I was told that I had cancer, I was told that I need not tell anyone. No one needed to know, the doctors told me. That seemed OK. I had respect and admiration for them. They knew what was right...or so I thought. But, within days, I found You nudging me to be free with the truth. Every inch of my being told me to tell of my disease. Somehow, in the midst of it all, You made me realize the good that would come from being open and honest. How I reacted to this terrible illness would help others see their own way more clearly.

While it wasn't the popular thing to do in 1978, I decided to speak openly. We were living in a time when society thought good things happened to good people and bad things happened to bad people. Those days are now behind us. We should not measure the worth of people by the good and bad that happens in their lives. Good and bad are not evenly distributed. The only thing we know for sure is that good and bad things do exist. We can celebrate both, knowing that You are always part of the celebration. Others see You in us. You confirm who You are through us.

Speak clearly to me so that I may, in turn, speak clearly to others. To work for Your good is my mission. Point me in the right direction. Open my eyes, my ears, and my mouth that I may see You more vividly, hear You more clearly, and speak of You more honestly. You walk the journey of illness with us just as You walk the journey of health. You like being along. Give me the good fortune never to leave You out of any area of my life. Without You, all is flat and meaningless.

Days of doubt are drab.
Days of silence are sad.
Days with no conversations with You give no comfort.
Days lacking You are lonely.
Days away from You cause anxiety.
Days without You are like the darkest of nights.

The pit of loneliness is real. The pit is deep and impossible. Never let me enter it. Keep me close to You. It is in being close to You that I get to know You. That closeness helps me to know You so that I might tell others of Your delightful ways.

Happier Person

A ray of sun,
   a salty tear,
   a clap of thunder,
   a drop of rain,
   a clover leaf,
   a summer storm,
   a heavy rock,
   a pebble of sand,
   a tree so tall,
   a leaf so green,
   a smiling face, and
   a helping hand
   touched me today.

My illness has made me
   a happier person.

Thank You, Lord.

Slowing Down

It's hard to slow down. My brakes work, but I don't use them often enough. Slowing down gives me time and space in my day for You, the You I long to know better and love more. Slow me down, Lord. Slow me down.

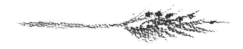

Embrace Me

Embrace me, O God. Help me to be calm and restful. Enhance my ability to listen. In the quiet of my life, You become vibrant and tender.

I pray that I might be direct with You. You lift my spirit. You have time for all of us. You are so predictable. I pray to be more like You. I receive many gifts from my illness because it is the direction that You have chosen to draw me to Yourself so that I might be of value to others. I pray that they may see You in me.

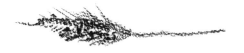

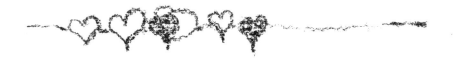

Holy Hearts

Like some finely tuned piece of machinery, I climbed onto the medical conveyor belt to health. Hundreds of people had led the way. I was to benefit from their bravery. I was to benefit from their courage. You know who they are. Will you thank them for me? I am grateful to them, especially for their ability to say yes even though the early procedures were experimental and the outcomes uncertain.

You gave them the strength to pave the way for us who were to follow. Blessed be their lives, for they were filled with meaning. They responded bravely that others who followed might benefit. Blessed be their spirit. Holy were their hearts.

University of Despair

Never permit me to enter the university of despair. It would be easy to give in.

Giving up would make those who love me unhappy. They have invested their love, their time, and their energy in supporting me. For their sakes, I must never give up. The very least I can do for all their kindness and prayer is to be grateful. Their hope is contagious.

I have the wonderful gift of bringing them happiness. I must hold on tightly to keep my spirits high. They deserve me at my best. The best I can be is important to my wellness. The chain of people who surround me is depending on me.

Will You never let despair enter my world, no matter

how difficult things may be? You and I will work together to battle even the least hint of giving up the fight. Never let me enter the university of despair.

♡ *Gladden the soul of your servant, for to you, O Lord, I lift up my soul.*

Psalm 86:4

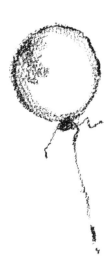

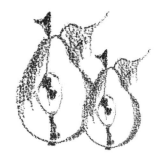

Savannah

Savannah was my friend. After being in an automobile accident, she went to an early grave. She was special in all sorts of ways. Recently, as I sat at her grave site, I was aware that our dry summer had left the grass and the earth unwatered. A slight mound in the ground marked the outline of the object that holds her earthly remains.

It was not like Savannah to be so quiet. Visions of her tiny four-foot, eleven-inch frame flashed before me. Her smile had always been contagious. Her spirit was full of You.

She gave us a beautiful Bible for our twenty-fifth wedding anniversary. Its soft leather cover, ribbons, and gold-edged onionskin pages made it an instant treasure.

How like Savannah to share the wonders of Your

Word with us! Savannah did all she did with confidence and determination. She would stop in the middle of any task if she thought she was needed. She always had time for her family and friends.

During my chemotherapy days, she would surprise us with delicious delights she had prepared in her kitchen. Our meals were not simply extensions of meals she prepared for her family. They were soft morsels that were agreeable to my damaged digestive system. It was easy to digest her carefully prepared treats.

She always had time for You. She lived in Your image. A day with Savannah was also a day with You. Didn't the three of us have joyful afternoons with one another? She rests now with You. I sit by her gravesite knowing for sure that the two of You are happy.

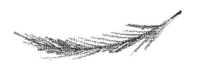

Fragile and Feather-Like

Fragile and feather-like I lie before You. Weak and worried I am by Your side. Will just being with You make me happy and healthy? What can I do to make things better? I must participate in the journey with You. Even when I am at my worst, I must point this fragile and feather-like creature towards wellness. Help me to realize that there are those more fragile, weaker, and more worried in this world. Today, I ask that we all join hands and walk together where we will meet happy and healthy as we once were, ready to help the fragile and the feather-like. Let us all lift our sights to You. Your Spirit from on high will float from above and fill our weaknesses and ease our worries.

My New Heart

You created my heart for me. When it wore out You found me a new one. You created my new heart for a young twenty-nine-year-old. Today I carry her heart for her. Have I thanked You lately for this miracle? Forgive me if I sometimes forget the bigness of what You have done for me. The heart transplant process was long and tedious. I wonder if I had known what was ahead, whether I would have done it? Of course, I would.

> You held my hand.
> You never left my side.
> You did not forsake me.
> You were always there for me.
> You were so sure things would be OK.

I never doubted because You never left me alone.

I was not lonely, frightened, nor anxious.

It was all such a mysterious adventure. I followed as You led the way. You gave me this experience that I might show others the strength and the resources we all have within us. Today I can look back with wonder and pride at the courage You gave me.

♡ *A glad heart makes a cheerful countenance, but by sorrow of heart the spirit is broken.*

Proverbs 15:13

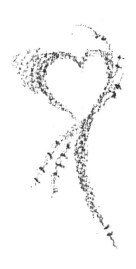

The Great Engineer

Yesterday the skilled, gentle hands of the gastroenterologist explored the area where my liver lies nestled under my rib cage. Quiet filled the small examining room. His eyes closed so that his sense of touch could be enhanced. Slowly and tenderly his hands moved around the area, exploring what has become a terrible source of pain. The bile duct seems not to want to do its job. The only mental picture I can conjure up is one of the liver and onions that Mother cooked so many years ago. I carry those childhood experiences with me. Today I realize the importance of this organ in my body.

The liver is seldom discussed or given much thought. Images of it aren't used like we use the images of the heart.

We "wear our heart on our sleeve." It sounds silly to say "I love you with my whole liver." But in reality, I have learned the liver is just as important as the heart. Without it, we would be in serious trouble.

Thank You for the marvelous way You designed us. I never cease to be amazed. You are the Great Engineer.

Please comfort my liver. Make it happy again. Let it work efficiently. Don't let it turn the whites of my eyes yellow nor my skin orange. You know how it was designed and constructed. You are the Great Engineer.

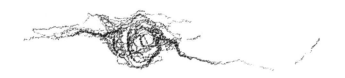

Just Humans

There are no tragedies in life if we know and love You. Sadness and hurt will always be part of our lives on earth. It is just part of being the simple humans we are. Our heavenly homes will know no sadness. You will be there. Saints will live among us. Let us treasure them. You have given us great wealth.

The faces all around us reflect You. Let us never forget to offer a smile to each of them.

I am sorry that there are those who do not know or who reject or who ignore You. They are the real losers in life.

When darkness falls, You seem to comfort me from above. Your presence is more real in the peace and quiet of night.

Today Is No Longer Yesterday

Today I don't feel quite right. I long for the life of long ago. Things were easier then. Coming and going and doing seemed easy and joyful. Energy filled my body. It only had to be turned on with the switch of a healthy starter.

Today is no longer yesterday. Gone are the things of a different time. They all seemed right and good. Sometimes I wonder, for today while I don't feel things are quite right, I realize the important things of life are far better than ever! Today I am full of the spirit of love.

See the invisible, Lord. Help me apply the Christian life to all of my life.

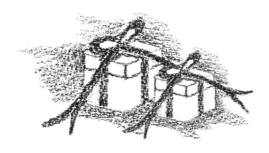

God's Gifts

I once thought I had to make a list of the things I did in a day. Now, I realize that list doesn't need to be filled with concrete things, things I could tell people if they asked, "What did you do today?"

No longer do those lists exist. Now, my days are filled with making memories…happy memories. I spent yesterday alone. I touched the leaves in my garden. I threw a bright yellow tennis ball to our big red, furry creation of God, our Irish setter named Peaches. I marveled at her joy in retrieving the ball.

The small, childlike brain in her chiseled head gave her small clues to where the ball had gone. Her need is to be happy, to give completely of herself. God created this wonder just for us to love. He wants us to be happy. He wants us to know love. Peaches never scolds me; she is always glad to see me. She is patient and peaceful. She is one of God's gifts to us.

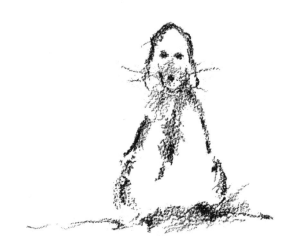

Joy in Illness

There is joy in illness. There are times when I cannot see it; at other times it is very obvious. The joy that I feel proves that You love me. It proves that I love You.

The proof is in the magic of Your gift. You suffered so much more than I ever will. There is joy found in the illness. The proof is in the magic of Your grace.

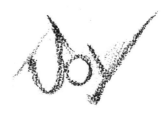

It Is Worth the Wait

He makes the wait worthwhile.
He makes the wait easy.

Waiting for God makes me smile.
It's easy to share the wait.

Waiting for God makes us long
for Him more and more.

Waiting for God
makes me patient.

The wait is filled with uncertainties
and even some doubts.

The wait is full of mystery.
The wait promises rewards.

I can hardly wait.
The wait excites me.

The wait is sure.
The wait goes on!

When the wait ends, all that is good begins.
It will all be worth the wait!

Spots of Loneliness

Since being very sick, there is loneliness deep within. You fill this loneliness. You fill me to the brim with Your Spirit. I am full of You.

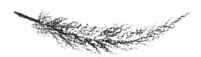

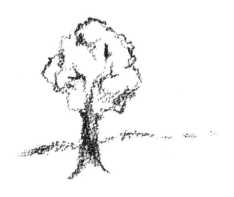

Good Things

The good things have always been. You shared so much of them with me. The good of illness has become my friend. It has silenced the noisy clamor of that other world in which I once lived.

Thank You, Lord.

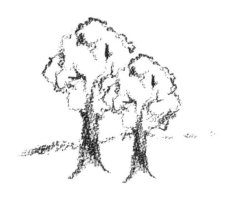

You Make Me Happy

O God, how happy You make me. You gave me ways to learn to pray. You helped me nourish our friendship. You showed me the way to You through the suffering of Your Son. My own suffering seems small in comparison. Help me to remember how He suffered and died so that I might live in You.

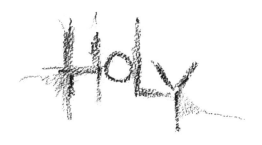

Aunt Annie Was Still

Recently I have learned the meaning of being still. For ever so long, stillness was new to me. My world was noisy. I have always talked too much. I have worked hard to be still. It is not always easy. Old behaviors are hard to change. However, once changed, we can rejoice.

My Great-Aunt Annie was quiet and always at peace. She lived in a room in Grandma Casey's house. She silently moved around the house. She cooked, cleaned, washed, and ironed. Every afternoon she sat in her chair in a ray of sunshine in the living room of the big, old house, saying her prayers.

As a child, I watched. Her lips moved as she silently read the words from her worn prayer book. My memory of her is clear. She had a mission. She ever so quietly moved closer to it each day. I work to be more like Aunt Annie. Being still and silent makes me strong.

♡ *And, let the peace of Christ rule in your hearts.*

Colossians 3:15

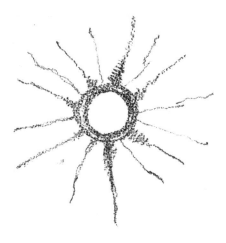

I Wonder

Sometimes I wonder who will read these prayers. I think long before I write. I don't want to waste Your time. I do not want to waste the time of my readers. My desire is to help them see meaning in their lives and accept You as:

Their friend

Their hope

Their love

Their comfort-giver

Their final solution

Their care-giver

Their peace-speaker

Their great savior

It is to You that I direct my attention. Teach me to talk to You.

On dry days, wet my spirits.

On sad days, shield me from myself.

On disorganized days, let me see order.

On rough days, smooth out the bumps.

On happy days, let me rejoice with You.

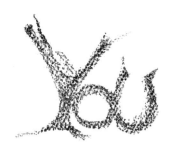

I Am So Small

Though I am so small,
You know and love me.

Thank You, Lord.

♡ *I lay down my life for the sheep.*

John 10:15

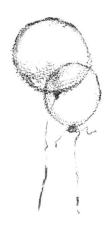

You Helped Me See the Way

You helped me see the way when the doctor told me I had cancer. You helped me hear what needed to be done to rid the cancer from by body. His words made sense. I was ready for more surgery. I understood how chemotherapy would kill the cancerous cells. The radiation I was to receive would center on the spot were the tumor once was. That beam of radiation would eradicate any cells that might have been left behind. Without it, those cells might reappear years from now. The way seemed easy. It had to be taken one day at a time. You were to join me on the journey. You helped me see the way.

As the chemotherapy entered my blood stream, the red liquid flowed into every inch of my body. Receiving chemotherapy was like traveling on rough water. You carried me through the choppy sea. It seemed easy with You along for the journey. The red liquid called Adriamycin was ugly. Out of the ugliness came happiness, for You did, indeed, carry me through that rough water.

When the heavy door of the radiation room closed and I was alone with that huge machine that I really never quite understood, You stood by me. The silence of the room, and then the clatter of the radiation machine, weren't as scary as they might have been because You were there.

You helped me see the reason that You never gave up hope. You taught me through Your example that hope was one of the most important parts of the puzzle to wellness. When I was well, the word *hope* was a small part of my vocabulary. Illness, disease, and all that accompanies them made the word *hope* gigantic!

Of the three virtues – faith, hope, and charity – that we learned so long ago, faith and charity seemed to be prime, but illness and suffering, pain and discomfort taught me the glories of hope. Hope gave me a look at tomorrow. Hope moved me from day to day. Hope helped me to see the bright side of the mountain. Hope made the climb out of terrible illness easier. You helped me not to give up hope ever. Whenever I could see the bright side of the mountain, I knew You were helping me to see the way.

♡ *A cheerful look brings joy to the heart; and good news gives health to the bones.*

Proverbs 15:30

Bus Stop

A lady alone, misshapen by her illness, waited patiently at the bus stop. When I asked if I could give her a lift she said, "Bless you, my child."

You rode in my car today.

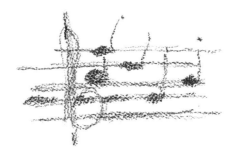

Loneliness

With illness comes loneliness. Loneliness is felt, not seen. It has no color. It has no shape. It has no form. It just is. To be lonely is to wish for meaning. My pain sets me apart from others. It sometimes keeps me from being able to interact. It keeps me inside myself. The hurt keeps my attention. It's lonesome inside. The feeling is real.

While it does not wave like a red flag or shriek like a fire alarm, it consumes a part of me that I once was. Help me work to regain that spirit where I can be outside myself, able to enjoy, to help, to interact with people around me. I want so much to be well enough to be able to tell others about You and to be more like You. If it is Your will, I want to sing and dance and write and paint again.

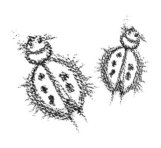

Bed Bugs

When mother put us to bed, she would always say, "Sleep tight. Don't let the bedbugs bite." We'd laugh and play like we were bedbugs, and, before we knew it, we were asleep. We awoke refreshed.

When the lights went out, I often wondered if You slept too. My childhood images were of You sleeping in a regal bed, tucked high into a puffy cloud with a fat comforter woven with threads of gold. My childlike reasoning made me think that You slept while I slept.

Our simple humanness makes it difficult to imagine the You that You are. How can You possibly be so real and loving? How can You take care of all of us? When do You have time to sleep? Will we need sleep when we are with You in Heaven?

Our earthliness is so limiting. Forgive me for even thinking to compare us to You. Of course, You don't need sleep. You are our God and our Protector. Of course You won't let the bedbugs bite.

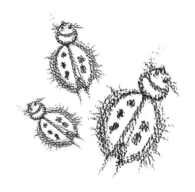

So Much To Say

When I was growing up, my best friend's name was Carole. We could talk for hours and hours. We had to whisper in class so as not to get scolded by our teachers. We had so much to say to one another, we had to write notes back and forth that we sneaked to one another so no one would catch us. We had so much to say, the days and evenings weren't long enough. Our nightly telephone conversations could have gone on forever if our mothers had not eventually put a stop to them. We were able to jabber on and on. There was so much to say.

In high school, my boyfriend's name was Mike. He and I would talk during our walk from the public square in Canton, Ohio, to the comer of 25th Street and Cleveland

Avenue. After twenty-five blocks of constant conversation, we would stand on the corner for another hour before we finally parted for our homes. There was just so much to say.

I met my husband in college. His name is Jerry. We could talk far into the hours of the night. There seemed no end to our conversations. Our letters to one another were pages long. There was so much to say.

Today, at 65, as I sit under my favorite palm tree on the beach in Naples, Florida, I observe people closely. Young teenagers like Carole and I or Mike and I wander up and down the beach talking. Their hands gesture as they share one story after another. Their never-ending chatter brings smiles to their faces.

Each day a small group of 60-year-olds sit in colorful beach chairs in a neat circle in the sand. As waves wash up on the beach in simple rhythm, these 60-year-olds speak with animation. They share stories and laughter. They start their visiting early in the day.

Two-by-two they leave their neat circle of friends to test the water. They compare how the water makes them feel. They laugh. They float. Their heads and their toes stick out above the water. All the time they talk.

At 4:30 they pack up their chairs, fold their towels, and reluctantly return to their vacation apartments. Obviously, they are sad to see their day of conversation come to an end. There is so much to say.

Someplace along the way, however, the cycle of communication, animation, and chatter seems to come to an end for some people. Beside me sits an elderly couple. They are bent. They wear sad and grumpy faces. They are silent. They stare into space. If a chair needs to be moved, she points, he responds.

Today she served him lunch from a plastic deli bag. Tuna sandwiches were softly munched. Potato chips crunched loudly. Diet Coke was swallowed in noticeable gulps. Their silence was deafening. There seemed to be nothing to say. I watch and I wonder.

Did they ever have so much to say to a grade school best friend that the day wasn't long enough? Did they ever stand on a street corner blocks from their homes, leaning against the street sign post, hating to part because there was so much still unsaid? Did they ever sit on a beach in a colorful chair exchanging the stories of their lives?

Have they run out of words? Does conversation become old as we get wrinkled and puckered? Has everything that needs to be said been said? Or, is there a chance that they never had much to say in the first place?

Just why does talking cease? Are there reasons for such long, sad silence? Could they be sick, depressed, worried? Could it be that growing has stopped?

Talk is healing. It is therapeutic. New thoughts and ideas begin conversation. Information brings with it wonderment. After reading a good book comes the tremendous urge to share its message.

Old is but a number of years. The years build mountains of memories. Change encourages exchanges.

Exchanges bring forth knowledge. Knowledge makes the search begin. The search starts the ideas. The ideas formulate the words. The words nurture the friendship.

Could it be that it all stops because there is no future? Hope has diminished. Time lingers. Sameness becomes commonplace. Boredom sets in. The exchange is over. Words dry up. Silence is now golden, like the years of people who live them.

Could it be that the relationship should never have been or has gone stale? Nothing new happens. Behavior is predictable. Breakfast, lunch, and dinner are served by the clock. New clothing isn't needed. The old hasn't worn out. There's nothing new in the grocery cart. Sameness becomes the enemy. Little joy exists. As the end nears is there no need to talk? Is there nothing about which to laugh?

Let us keep the tank of talk on full. Reading, writing, learning, thinking, questioning, remembering, challenging, all bring with them a steady flow of exchange, knowledge, searching, and friendly, stimulating conversation.

Why not begin each day by saying good morning to God? He loves to hear your voice. Then call a good friend, and be a good listener. The art of conversation includes the very important ingredient – listening. Maybe your friend needs someone with ears that work. Try a friendly hello to someone in the grocery store. That person might live alone, and the sound of your voice is a gift. Search out a child or two with whom to commune. What a joyful experience that can be!

Sit quietly, and softly talk to your cat or dog. Repeat endearing words they have come to understand. They will be grateful, and they will respond in their own ways. Find a pet store with a parrot. You'll be sure to get an answer after asking any silly question.

Ask questions of those you love. Repeat, in question form, the last part of what they say. It will be fascinating how they will tell you more and more of what is on their mind. You show you care about them when you listen and respond.

Turn off the television. Those people aren't talking with you, they are talking at you.

End each day with a prayer to our Lord. Thank Him for all the glories of the day and for the gift of gab. He loves to talk with you. If you listen very carefully, you may hear His joyful words. Then there will be so much to say.

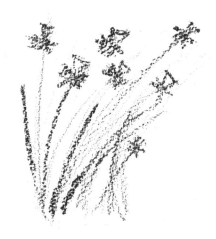

Happy Birthday, Jesus

Today is your birthday, Jesus. The television and radio tell of snowflakes, Bethlehem, a manger, a silent night, a star in the sky, angels singing, and a savior who is Christ the Lord.

They also tell of Santa, a reindeer with a red nose, bargains galore, decorated trees in every home, and traffic jams.

Mixed messages in this mixed-up world of ours. Your birthday is very special. It brings with it the promise of our salvation. You came as a beautiful baby to show us how to live. You told us through Your word how to live. From Your plain, simple childhood emerged a graceful, quiet, young adult. You went about Your father's business. Using parables, miracles and concrete situations, You clearly directed us. Ours is only to listen, learn, and follow.

We hope this is a happy birthday for You. Look down on us in love and compassion. We are often out of step. We sometimes seem confused, yet we stab at attempting to do all things in Your name.

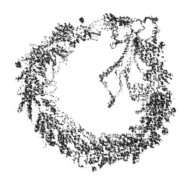

I Wait, I Wander, and I Wonder

I wait and I wander,
looking for Your sweet words.

I wait and I wander,
looking for Your strong voice.

I wait and I wonder,
Will this time of pain pass?

I wait and I wonder,
Will today pass?

I wait and I wonder,
Will a better tomorrow ever come?

I wait and I wander,
expecting a better day.

I wait and I wonder,
Will You come to me?

I wait and I wonder,
Am I missing Your healing grace?

I wait and I wonder,
Will I ever be well again?

I wait as I grow in You;
it gets easier and easier.

I wonder as I wander with You,
How much more is there to learn?

♡ *When, at night, I cry out in your presence, let my prayer come before you; incline your ear to my cry.*

Psalm 88:1–2

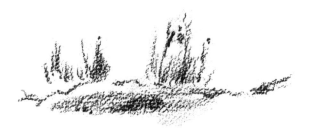

I Am Not Angry

The remnants of yesterday fall to the ground, broken and crumpled. My healthy body is no more. The remains and scars of serious illness have taken away some of the things of the world.

I am not sad.

I am not angry.

I am not resentful.

I am not disappointed.

I am cheerful.

I am calm.

I am relaxed.

I am lighthearted.

I am grateful.

Today I know You. I know for sure there is a purpose to my illness, my pain, and my suffering. I herald the coming of the end of this earthly life that it might end in serenity with You at my side.

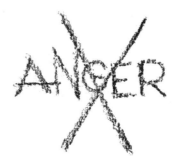

Will I Be Prepared?

Your suffering and death were perfect, nothing needed. Your last cry in John's gospel is, "It is finished." We are so joined to You that our sufferings continue the work of salvation. We can share in it. Remember each day that pain and illness allow us to live freely in joy and sorrow knowing that they are joined with the work of our Lord. Hence, the value of our suffering. We do not search for such; we are not masochists, but it makes pain productive. Our society has lost the value of suffering. Many try to run away into drugs or sex or alcohol. The list goes on and on. However, there is really no escape; no one leaves this world alive.

I will miss my world, my husband, my family and friends, the things of this plentiful place. As people of faith, we will all meet again. Our Irish setter, Peaches, and our silver shorthaired cat, K.C., and the joys of this earth will surely join us in unison with You, Father, Son, and Holy Spirit, to live together in love and peace. The turmoil of our earthly lives will be gone.

An exciting party lies ahead. You have made the plans, You have thought of every detail; the party will be no surprise. You will greet Your guests as they arrive. You have sent out the invitations; we need only to respond. You will decide when we will join You and Your loved ones. I wait patiently. When You need me, help me to make sure I am prepared.

I want to help plan the party. I will be like Martha. I will do the work. Just knowing that You are in the next room will be OK. I also want to be like Mary of Bethany and sit at Your feet, listening to Your preparations. Prepare me for my role in Your plans.

♡ *Be gracious to me, O Lord, for to you do I cry all day long.*

Psalm 86:3

Tommy's Angel Pushed Him

Seldom do I wish to be a young child again. I am very contented being the age I am. There is, however, one thing from my youth that I miss. And, it's that uncontrollable, "make-your-body-shake-all-over" laughter. It was laughter like no other, brought on by the silliest of things.

"Church laughter" was sometimes the best. We sat close together on the pews with our shoulders touching, and then, out of the blue, someone would start to laugh. It was contagious. It traveled up and down the pew, one to another. It was like yawning or coughing.

Once we started, a tap on the shoulder from our teacher or parent would only make it worse. It was hard for us to contain ourselves. It was difficult to take in a breath for fear that some big giggle would escape loudly from us, and we knew from experience that would only make things worse.

It would be hard to guess just what event from childhood brought on the best laughter. I think, however, a consistent, "sure-to-happen" laughing event happened in the fourth grade.

Tommy O'Brien was an adorable child with a round, innocent face. He seemed to stop growing vertically and continue to grow horizontally.

Our fourth grade teacher was very round, not young, and usually tired. Climbing the stairs to our second-floor classroom five times a day left her winded and wheezing.

She had developed the perfect discipline technique. She insisted that we sit on the very side of our seats in order that we leave room for our guardian angels. We were told that they were there to help us and to make us behave. We even named them. My angel's name was Lily. Sometimes we had to be silent in order that they could talk with one another. Occasionally, even today, I find myself unconsciously sitting on the edge of my chair, leaving room for the now-very-old Lily.

One day, during quiet time, which sometimes lasted all day, there was a terrible thud in the classroom. It scared us. Tommy O'Brien flew from his seat onto the floor. We were startled. Then we heard him yell, "She pushed me!"

Sister commanded him to get up from the floor: "Get up immediately, Mr. O'Brien!"

"She pushed me! My guardian angel pushed me! She's

getting so fat there isn't room on the seat for both of us any-more!"

"Get up!" Sister yelled.

"Not until you tell her not to push me again!" Tommy responded.

Even today, the picture of our round and tired teacher disciplining Tommy's guardian angel makes me want to laugh.

Tommy had found an ingenious way to break Sister's once-perfect discipline code. Tommy had found a way to bring joy into our otherwise dull days. Because of the positive peer response, Tommy's falls to the polished wooden floor became more frequent.

Never again were we bored. We always knew that, at the right time, Tommy would bring life to our class. The laughter prompting the event was always unexpected and unpredictable. Sometimes we were sure it would never happen again when, out of the blue, there he was sprawled on the floor shaking his finger in mid-air, scolding his over-weight guardian angel.

Poor Sister had lost complete control of us, and she knew it. She threatened to take our guardian angels away from us. We knew that was not in her power. She tried everything; once she told us that the guardian angels were all sick and had to stay in heaven all day. She needed just one day when she could be sure Tommy would stay in his seat. Tommy didn't believe angels got sick. While the rest of us sat on the middle of our seats that day, Tommy hung from the side of his seat. His angel was with him. Sister saw her plea hadn't worked.

I often wonder where Tommy O'Brien is today. Is he still making people delight in laughter?

Yes, those youthful days were filled with that uncontrollable, "make-your-body-shake-all-over" laughter that continues to be the best!

Your Child

I like being Your child. While I am but a speck as You look down, You know every hair on my head and freckle on my face. You have known me forever. You never faltered in Your love for me. At times, I have not deserved Your love or Your tenderness. You stay by my side in spite of my earthly wanderings.

When I wandered, You found me.

When I worked, You reached out to me.

When I drifted, You kept me tethered to your side.

When I ventured far from You, You waited with Your arms outstretched for my return.

You gave me the love for which I longed. You removed the scars caused by my wanderings and made me clean and whole again. I live in You. I like being Your child.

Patience

Patience is the virtue I work to make strong. Help me be quiet in my suffering. Complaining to others only makes them feel anxious and helpless.

All I have to give to others is my attitude about illness and pain. Keep a smile on my face that I might radiate the goodness I know from You.

Intellect and will are what You gave me to quiet the hurt from within. I am able to reason, to learn, and to accept my pain.

Never allow me to feel angry or to pity myself. I will never question Your ways. You are my Lord and my God. In You I put my trust.

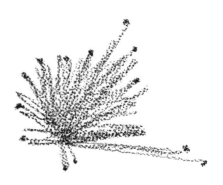

Light of Hope

The white light that surrounds and protects us is You. With determination and tenacity, I keep within that light. It is there as sure as life. It glows as it travels with me. It is the light of hope, hope that I may love You more with the passing of each day. That light of hope helps to snuff out the pain. Pain is what helps to make things real. Layered front to back and top to bottom, I am aware of who I am, who I really am, and who You are, who You really are. I am not as close to You without pain. Your reasons become clear to me. Each day I work to be close to You. I want to move away from earthly things. They no longer are meaningful. I move inside myself. I like looking out at the world. Removing the clutter makes it easier to be with You in the light of hope.

O, Great Listener

O great listener, please help me to tolerate the damage done to my bones that the newly diagnosed osteoporosis is causing. The crushing of my rib cage makes it difficult for me to eat and to stand. My chest feels like a baby elephant is standing on it. Along with being uncomfortable, it is very painful. Please hear my plea for some relief. Please make the discomfort tolerable. Please slow down the deterioration process.

Jerry is concerned. The worry shows in his face. I hate being a worry to him. Help us. Your way is our way. We will be patient. We will accept reality, no matter how severe it becomes.

Bless my broken bones. Bless my crushed frame.

Though it is bent and crippled, I will accept its gradual deterioration. I pray that others like me will be given the grace to tolerate the sadness that comes with a changing body. Bone pain is new to me. Teach me to learn to live peacefully in spite of it. In all things, I hold true to You. Thank You for listening.

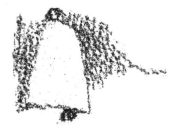

Our Heavenly Home

Our home with You and all Your saints will never need repair. Its windows will shine with Your love. Its door will swing freely. Its roof will touch the stars. Its walls will be strong. We will be forever content in the perfection You have planned for us. Make clear my path to Your door. I will knock, and You will answer, "Hello Friend!"

You are my treasure; I long to keep You by my side.

Your gentleness softens this tough world.

You always wait for me.

You are never angry when I put less important things first.

There are no bad times when You are near.

The nearer You are the happier I am.

With You by my side I can do anything.
There is good all around us. You show us where to look.
The search is simple.
We just have to learn to listen to that soft whisper.
In You there is all there ever needs to be.

♡ *Blessed are the poor in spirit, for theirs is the kingdom of Heaven.*

♡ *Blessed are those who mourn, for they will be comforted.*

Matthew 5:3–4

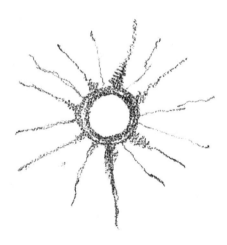

Visions

Visions of death dance gracefully before us. Leaving this earth will be simple, for You will have us ready to join You in the heavenly home You have prepared for us. Oh, I so hope that You will be happy to see us. We will dance and sing and walk the meadows of joy. The journey will be never-ending. Illness and pain and suffering will be no more. Thank You for my illness for it has given me an appreciation for how much You want me with You.

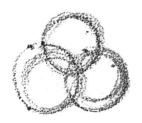

God Is

God is under every stone,
reachable, omnipresent, and everywhere.

God is ours, yours, truth,
alive, and never vague.

God is curious, zestful, simple,
all-knowing, and immovable.

God is delightful, powerful,
restful, cheerful, happy, and wonderful.

God is all, abundant, great,
quiet, and good.

God is first, bright, warm,
open, and friendly.

God is artistic, athletic,
youthful, creative, and Master.

God is in the Trinity:
Father, Son, and Holy Spirit.

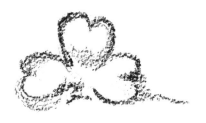

A Happy Lot

We live in an almost perfect community. Our city works at being a kind place. We seem to be centered in You. Love thy neighbor as thyself permeates our paths. Love for one another is obvious.

We recognize our differences and admire those differences. We take joy in our similiarities. Like the contents of a new box of crayons, we stand shoulder to shoulder, respecting one another. We reach out to one another. We need one another. Our love for one another is apparent in the smallest of gestures. People stop to allow others to cross in front of them. Complete strangers run to the aid of someone in distress.

It is obvious that we are a community with You at our

core. We share what we know and love about You with one another. Hurt, gossip, and unkindness are rare. We help one another to resist falling into ugly patterns. The more we grow in community with You, the happier and holier we become.

Your Spirit rests in us, keeping us always on guard. Bless us as we work to stay in Your word and struggle to be more like You. For, with You in our midst, a happy lot are we.

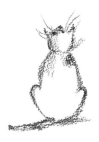

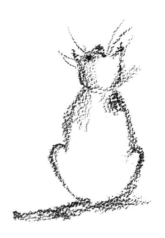

A Cat Speaks Out

I often sit here wondering how they found me. I was born in a cattery. There were many of us. We all looked alike. My first recognition of my Mom and Dad was how beautiful they both were. Their silver fur tipped with black was perfectly designed. They were exact duplicates. Dad weighed ten pounds, and Mom was a tiny little six pounds. My sister and I loved them very much. They were obviously proud of us. We were such happy babies.

Mom taught us how to wash behind our ears and how to clean our beautiful silver fur. Dad taught us how to use our litter box. Before long, we were separated from Mom and Dad and placed in a big cage-like room. It was called a cattery.

I often think about that big cage. Some of my relatives had been there for years. The boys were called studs by our caretakers. Now and then they would be taken out of the big cage to "meet a new girlfriend." I never quite understood what that was all about. I can remember how, every now and then, someone with big, strong hands would pick me up. She would hold me close to her face. She would examine me carefully. "You're going to make a good one," she would tell me. "A good what?" I wondered.

Long, boring months rolled by. My sister and I stuck together. We felt like strangers among all those big ones just like us. We often meowed together. We couldn't figure out why we were there. We just sat, slept and once a day a big hand reached in a door. Several bowls of dry, crunchy things that smelled good were placed on the floor. Everyone else got to them first. We were tiny and couldn't fight our way to the front. There was almost always some left for us.

Every now and again those big hands would gather up several of my relatives that were especially big and beautiful. They were given what the big-handed person called a bath. Terrible screeching came from a room nearby. They always smelled funny when they returned to the big cage. The next day they would disappear again. This time they seemed to be gone forever, taken away in little carrying cases with open circles around the sides.

After a very long time, they would return. Their tired faces greeted us. The people who took them would say nice things as they returned the beauties to our cage, things like, "special" and "real winners." They hung blue ribbons on our big cage-like room. Those travelers got lots of attention after a "blue ribbon day." Late at night, when everything was quiet, the tired travelers would tell us about their time away. They had been to what they called a "cat show." They were held up in the air, and stretched out by a person called a judge. People sat in chairs and looked admiringly at them. Now and then the audience would "ooh" and "ahh."

Life didn't seem much fun for them or for us. What was this all about? We had the urge to be free. All this seemed unnatural. We needed to be loved. We thought there should be more to life than this.

One grim day, when I was about five months old, the lady with the big hands looked closely at my private parts. "What? One didn't drop," she told a tall man who stood very close to us. He too examined me.

"What hadn't dropped?" I wondered.

The next thing I knew I was in a big tub of warm water. Smelly suds covered my lovely clean fur. I had learned to care for myself. "Whatever was she doing to me?" I wanted to screech at the top of my lungs. Then warm air shot out the end of a tube of some sort of plastic machine. She rubbed me with an ugly, worn, pink towel. She fluffed me.

And then, the next day I was off with my relatives to one of those cat shows. I couldn't wait. "Would I return with one of those big blue ribbons to hang on the outside of the cattery?" I hoped I would. Then I'd get the attention those who won blue ribbons always got. I kissed my sister good-bye.

They must have had other plans for her.

Traveling for the first time in a tiny box with round open air holes along the sides was new to me. I could peek out. Things looked enormous and frightening through the holes. Every once in a while, a huge finger poked through one of the holes. I wanted to swat at it but didn't trust what might happen. I decided it was smarter just to try to cope. The blue ribbon loomed in my mind. Wow! I could hardly wait!

There were hundreds of us at the cat show. I never thought there were so many of us. Some of the others were big. One big cat was called a Maine Coon. He scared me to death. No way I could get a blue ribbon if I had to be held up beside him. Some of them even had blue eyes. They cried like babies.

My little red bed from home was placed in a small cage. It was nice watching the people walk by. People looked in at me. Their faces nearly touched the bars on the cage. They read aloud a sign the tall man had hung on the door of my cage. I heard them say, "Five-month-old Classic Silver American Shorthair for sale." "For Sale?" I wondered what that meant. Would I get a blue ribbon if I "sailed?"

Several times I was scooped from the cage. People looked at me closely. They smiled nicely. They liked me. Then they would pull up my tail and say "Oh, only one dropped." There it was again. Something hadn't dropped.

What in heaven's name were they looking for? No, nothing had dropped; I examined the floor closely.

My relatives were carried away in the arms of the big, tall pair. They returned. More blue ribbons. When was it going to be my turn? The afternoon was long. I was tired. My eyes were half closed. I felt terrible. I hadn't used my litter box for several days. I felt sick.

From across the room a big, kind-faced man looked right at me. I barely heard him say to the energetic lady who was with him, "Look at that cat!" Quickly they came across the room. They asked if they could hold me. Oh, it felt good to be held by such loving hands. Sweetly they looked into my face. The nice lady whispered into my ear. It was love at first sight. They liked me, and I liked them. They never even bothered to look under my tail. They seemed not to care about that thing that had not dropped.

By this time, I knew I was sick. Oh, how I wanted to feel free. I needed water. I was exhausted. It had been a tiring day. I had been poked, stared at, held, neglected, rejected, and I had never gotten to try to get one of those big blue ribbons.

Both of the nice people took turns holding me. They put me in their carrying case. Away we went. Oh, it was good to get out of that terrible place. The room had a strong cat smell. Some of those cats must not have been taught to be careful to always use their litter box and always, always, always, cover it up with litter.

"Why hadn't their dads taught them better? Mercy!"

Feeling sick, but glad to be away from the tall, big pair, I was placed on the back seat in my carrying case. They glanced back at me often. They seemed so happy. I wished I felt better. I probably would have enjoyed the trip more.

The car stopped. I had been napping. The carrier moved. I peeked out one of the circular holes. A friendly looking, brown house awaited us. They unlocked a door. Once inside, they put the carrier on the floor and opened the top covering. I raised my tired head. Oh, dear. I could have cried when I saw the room. There were no bars, there was no cage. I was free. They stood silently as they watched with admiring eyes. I jumped out of the box. Ever so carefully, I sniffed around.

They showed me a pan of litter. I couldn't use it. Something was wrong down there. How would I ever tell them? Would they notice?

After a little water and food, I was permitted to fend for myself. Exhausted, I found a safe place under a bed. All that freedom at once was more than I could take. Sleep came easily.

Early the next morning, I was scooped up and put back into the carrying case. "Oh, no, what had I done wrong? Were they taking me back to the cattery?"

It was a short car ride to a place that smelled really funny. A man in a white coat looked through my fur. "No fleas," he stated. "No ear mites." Of course there were no fleas or ear mites. I had had that awful bath the night before. Then he did it. The inevitable happened again. He looked under my tail. "Oh dear, one hasn't dropped." There we were again on that subject.

The nice lady looked at the kind man. "Why didn't you notice that?" she asked him. "That was your area to check. What would I know about that?" she asked. He said he never really noticed. They shrugged. It didn't seem to matter to them, whatever it was.

The man in the white coat thought I had a temperature. "Probably a kidney infection," he thought. Boy, was I ever glad he discovered why I hadn't been able to use my litter box.

Back home we went. I think they were going to keep me. They gave me some pills. I was able to use my litter box. I ate a bowl of the most wonderful, moist, tasty food they forked from a tiny can with a green label into a special dish that said "pussy cat" on the front in big blue letters.

Within days I had roamed around the entire house. I could sleep anywhere I wanted. In the mornings, the sun warmed the soft velvet chairs in the dining room. In the afternoons, I found a basket with a little, three-degree heating pad in it. It warmed my tired body. In the evenings I sat on laps. We watched television together.

I never did get one of those blue ribbons at the cat show. I got something much, much better. I got myself two blue ribbon people who simply love me to death. I have always wondered and hoped that my dear, sweet little sister had the luck I had.

The months rolled by quickly. Whatever I wanted, I got. I spent a few days with the man in the white coat. He made me very sleepy, and when I awoke he told the nice lady he had gone in and removed the thing that had never dropped. Wow! I was glad that subject was closed!

Just when I had decided that life was perfect, something was added to our little perfect group of three. One warm summer afternoon, a big, red, long-legged, furry animal, which I later learned was a dog, arrived. She had big floppy ears and a cold wet nose. She licked me. "Oh no, a Dog! How could these nice people ruin what I had grown to know as perfection?" She was big and uncoordinated. She had no manners. She had no litter pan. She made terrible mistakes. Gradually things improved. The nice people seemed to like her. If they liked her, and they liked me, then I decided to learn to like her.

Today, we sit together. Her big, hot, red body keeps me warm. She answers when they call her Peaches. They tell people she's an Irish setter. She never did get a litter box. She goes to the door several times a day. Her litter pan must be outdoors.

To this day, I wonder how they ever found me. "Where would I be without them? I love them very much. Life is good. Life now has meaning. And to think they like me even though I never got one of those blue ribbons."

I look to them for love just as they look to You for Your love. I know love…they know love.

We Whisper Our Sorrows

While I dream of my heavenly destination, the mystery of how it all happens is frightening. Please give me the strength to be unafraid. Let me come to You relaxed and at peace. When my eyes close for the last time here on earth, let them open to the beauty of Your face.

Reach out Your hand that I may take hold of it. Pull me up to the heaven You have promised us. I pray that I will be ready to open my eyes to the wonder of it all. Let those who have gone before me await my arrival.

I will be glad to see them, especially those who have been my cancer pals on earth. Like some large sorority or fraternity, we have known the same suffering. In our groups, we have gathered to give one another courage and strength.

Hand in hand, with heads bowed, we have spoken in unison that You might hear us. With bald heads from chemotherapy, burned skin from radiation, and scars and incisions from surgery, we have shouted, and we have whispered our sorrows. You are in control of our destinies.

♡ *Blessed are you who weep now, for you shall laugh.*

From the writings of Luke

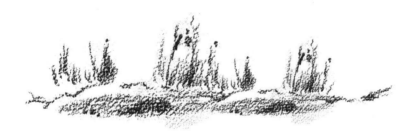

Shouts of Joy

We shout at ball games.
We shout at recess time.
We shout when we see a friend far off.

We shout when we are fearful.
We shout when we are joyful.
We shout when we need help.

We shout when we think we might drown.
We shout to get attention.
We shout to seek approval.

We shout when we are in need.
We shout to reinforce what we need.
We shout when we hurt.

We shout in the night,
 thinking that darkness stifles our sounds.
We shout on the beach
 so that the waves do not drown out
 our feeble sounds.
We shout in the rain
 so that the drops will not silence our words.

We shout to be heard.
Lord, hear our shouting.
We need Your love, Your strength,
 Your words of encouragement.

Hear us, O Lord. Hear our shouts.

♡ *On the day I called, you answered me; you increased my strength of soul.*

Psalm 138:3

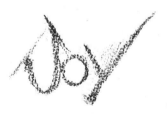

The Voiceless Listen

Help me to be voiceless. When I am quiet, I rest with You. You cradle me in Your warmth. You show me the way. You encourage me to share my bumps, and to be quiet when it hurts the most. In voicelessness, there is beauty. The beauty of the harmony we share quickly sheds light on the joys of knowing You.

The simple spark of prayer leads me to You. I wait anxiously to see You, to laugh with You, to help You do Your work. What a huge task You have! Like simple children we exist. You know and love us all. However do You do that?

You know our fingerprints and every detail of our bodies, our minds, and our hearts. We are Yours. You know and love us. Help me to bear up through this illness. Cancer is frightening. People don't know what to say. Some people move away. You stay near. Your nearness is obvious. It removes my fears. It makes me speechless. I pray this day that all of us on earth may find a way to listen more carefully to each other and to You.

For in this voicelessness, there is peace. In this voicelessness, there is no fear. In this voicelessness, I learn to listen.

♡ *May your kindness, O Lord, be upon us who have put our hope in you.*

Psalm 33:3

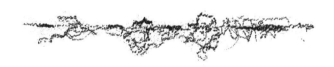

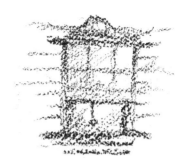

And Then She Flew Out the Window

Stories are told and retold. When I was a child, some of my favorite stories were those that my mother would tell of things my older sister did as a child.

Mary Ann is four years older than me. She was an independent, sure-of-herself child who was unpredictable, demanding, and difficult. She could dream up the most bizarre things to do before anyone ever thought them possible. It's hard for me to decide which of the wild tales to share with you. Our mother entertained us by the hour, for years with tale after tale.

The summer of 1936 was hot and steamy. I was just six months old. My mother and father had their hands full. Mary Ann had not enjoyed being dethroned and had become worse than she was as an only child. To relieve my parents of some of the stress and work, Grandma and Grandpa helped to care for Mary Ann. Aunt Mary, Mother's older sister and a fifth grade teacher, lived with Grandma and Grandpa in a large, three-story, white frame house on Louisiana Avenue, which sat high on a hill. A low, lush, rock garden filled the hill that led up to the house. The house was surrounded by lovely wisteria, small pussy willow trees, forsythia, and especially beautiful large white hydrangea bushes. We joyfully referred to them as "snowball bushes." Hollyhocks dotted the areas between the bushes.

Grandpa had taken all the proper precautions to make the house safe for the frequent visits of "the tyrant" as they had come to call Mary Ann. Locks were put on cupboards. Anything breakable or valuable was hidden away or stored up high. The moment "the baby" arrived for the day, the mantle in the living room looked like a mirage of sundry pieces of glass and family treasures lined up and protected from what was sure to be a quick and easy demise.

All the window screens had hooks all the way around their four sides "just in case." In the eaves of the house next door, a nest of baby robins poked their long, skinny necks high in the air waiting for their mother to bring them food.

Grandpa mowed the lawn around the hydrangea bushes, and Grandma said her afternoon prayers in the "baby's room," as "the baby" napped. At the sound of the phone, Grandma went to Aunt Mary's room to answer its ring. So as not to wake the baby, she whispered into the phone to my mother, who was on the other end of the line.

"The baby" woke up. (She was probably only pretending to sleep.) Clad only in a diaper and socks with high, white, laced shoes, she awakened, went to the window, and pulled herself up onto the 8" high baseboard that was in houses in those days. With her finely tuned dexterity, she carefully unhooked all the little hooks Grandpa had installed. She then "flew" out the window. She would later explain that she merely wanted to fly over to the house next door to visit the baby birds.

Much to Grandpa's surprise, she landed in the hydrangea bush smack in front of his hand-pushed little mower. Grandma heard his plea for help and yelled into the phone in her heavy Irish brogue, "Oh my God, be glory, she's flown out the window!" and immediately fainted, leaving my mother on the other end of the line, several miles away, begging for some explanation. This was the part of the story I always liked the best.

Mother would become animated and talk into an imaginary phone saying "Who flew out the window? Did "the baby" fly out the window? Oh my God in Heaven! Sweet Mother!" Grandma in her speechless faint lay on the floor. The trauma of it all thrilled me.

Mary Ann would sit smugly listening to the story. She had been through it. We knew the ending. Mother, Grandma, Grandpa, and Aunt Mary were sure Mary Ann was lying dead among the snowball bushes. But, as luck would have it, her heavy white shoes had weighted her properly so that she dropped feet first into the forever-after-worshiped hydrangea. The only mishap was a broken leg, which left her right foot a size smaller than her left foot. Every time we bought new shoes, the salesman had to hear the fly-out-the-window story. Everyone in the shoe store heard the story because "the tyrant" needed two sizes of shoes.

Never do I see a puffy snowball bush that I don't think of the excitement of that hot summer day of 1936 when I was only six months old. I have heard the story so many times, it's as if I were there. Telling and retelling stories can be such fun. Let us not allow e-mail, the computer, or any of our fast-moving inventions of today change one of the most joyful parts of our lives – the passing of stories, one generation to another, of the colorful, wonderful past.

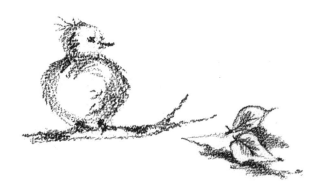

Please Take the Pain Away

The pain I have is real. It hurts. How hurtful Your pain must have been. It makes mine small in comparison.

I am so human that I can't seem to move away from the pain.

I try to put it second to everything, yet it fights to be first. It gets bigger and more constant.

No Time

God knows no time
    for boasting,
    for envy,
    for fear,
    for anger,
    for laziness,
    for pride,
    for cruelty,
    for lustfulness,
    for gluttony,
    to ask silly questions,
    for trivia.

God only has time for me, us, him, her, them.
All His time he devotes entirely to us.

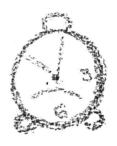

Let It Be Your Way

Let me be filled with Your love.
Let me never stop loving You.

Let me be at peace.
Let me be tranquil.

Let me be of help to others.
Let me be patient.

Let me hear You.
Let me learn from You.

Let me not enter into despair.
Let me be happy.

Let me see goodness in all things.
Let me free myself of things that separate us.

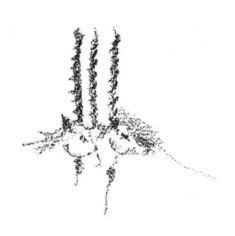

Merry-Go-Round

My life revolves around You. Round and round, like the carousel I so loved as a child. Its musical circles delighted my childhood spirit. You, the musical center of my life, revolve around me today. The sound of Your laughter makes me smile.

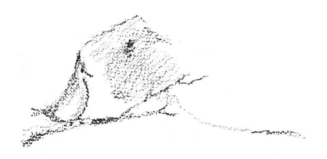

Nudge Me

Are You sure I am headed in the right direction? Give me a nudge should I start to stray.

I pray that all that I do is done in Your name. May people see You in me without my saying a word. May my every move, my very being show my love for You.

The things of this world are simple. They mean so little in comparison to the things of eternity. Help us to be constantly aware of this.

Make sure I do not let myself get caught in the hustle of earthly searching. You are the answer. Thank You for showing me the way to You. Keep me focused on You. Don't let me get distracted from You.

I Can Endure

Pain surrounds me. Inside and out it consumes me. How bad will it get? How long will it last? Will the doctors ever find the reasons for the pain? What is its source? Will it get bigger as the night grows? Front and back, it moves and then it connects. What will soften it? What can I say to explain it? To numb it would only shut it down temporarily. What about tomorrow? How many others are there this night who know pain personally? Do they reach out to You for help? Help them first, if You must. I can wait. I can endure.

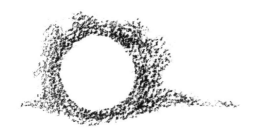

Change My Range

In this life, we can hold onto the old, which isn't going to stick around forever, or we can accept and welcome new into our lives. Whether we want to or not, we need to stay with it. Accept change. Move on.

Records went from 78s, to 45s, to 33⅓s, to 8-track, to tapes, and then CDs. Now, we can get music from the satellite.

We once rolled up our car windows by hand, shifted gears, and froze as the little heater box on the passenger side of the car heated only that passenger. Family talking and singing were replaced by AM, FM, speakers, disks, and tapes.

Our oven stopped working several weeks ago, My

husband went shopping for a new one. I stayed home. How different could a new oven be?

He returned from his first shopping venture with a new dishwasher! A dishwasher? Yes, the old one was on its last leg, I was informed.

The next trip to the appliance store brought a new range. The old one was electric; the new one is gas. Gas? Yes, people are cooking with gas today, I was reminded. Our mothers cooked with gas!

Finally, the oven arrived. A black, airplane-cockpit-like panel that is entirely digital is neatly situated above the new, black, streamlined doors. There are no knobs, no dials – just buttons and windows.

Innocently, within three short weeks, my kitchen changed. Things I once did automatically now take new plans, new cooking times, and new settings.

The new beauties in my kitchen seem to smile at me. They are friendly enough. What began with one worn oven has escalated into a technological maze. I stand among my new friends a bit apprehensive. I try not to show my feelings.

My dishwasher does so much more than "wash." It comes alive with the touch of a button. I expect an arm with a scrub brush to reach from it to scrub the floor. The range snaps on the heat. When it's off, it's off. There is no slow, gradual cooling.

Adjusting to change is part of staying on the escalator of life. Change is growth, and we remain young when we grow by accepting and welcoming new into our lives.

Love

God is love.
God is lovable.
God is loving.
God is lovely.

God is in love with us.
God knows how to love us.
God knows how to show love.
God knows how to share love.

God understands love.
God gives love because God is love.
God is the love of our lives.
God knows us beyond our imaginations.

God is LOVE.

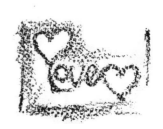

The Center of It All

Experience is the foundation of learning. Through the experience of having a heart transplant I have learned much. The old, big, floppy heart that was once firmly planted within my chest is now gone. It has been replaced with a tiny new heart, a heart taken from the body of a young lady. She was just twenty-nine years old.

Look what she did for me. Look at the gift she gave me. How do I share the immensity of the experience with her? All that I have learned from her generosity is immeasurable. My worn-out old heart is gone. It sits in a jar on a shelf in a research laboratory. A tiny new one replaces the enlarged, ragged, old one. Skilled hands prepared the open spot, and the healthy new heart was placed in its new home. Out with the old, in with the new. It only took four hours!

Overwhelmed, confused, not knowing the outcome, I moved on. Emily's heart became mine. She and I would experience life together from now on. We would know one being. From one huge experience, I became whole. From our becoming one, I found health. Emily and I learned to co-exist. As I wait, Emily pumps. Is she I? Am I she? Is life together compatible?

Life together is life with You. You found us struggling. You gave us new life. I long to meet Emily someday that I might thank her personally. You care for us now. Young Emily lives with You. Her earthly stay was short. You took her to You. She left behind her healthy heart that I might continue to give You glory on this earth. As believers, we will someday be together.

I delight in being at peace with what You do. While I don't always understand, I try not to control or foresee. I try to stay in Your center of love and attention.

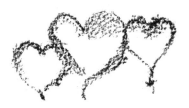

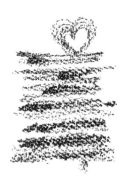

Layers of Love

The layers of Your love grow taller and taller. They combine to reach high into the space outside me. As the layers of love build, they lean a little to the left and back again to the right. The space between the layers narrows as the layers get higher and higher. The spaces are squeezed by the weight of love as it grows. Your love knows no boundaries.

No height is too high.

No width is too wide.

No length is too long.

No weight is too heavy.

The load of love from You is larger than life. Help me to layer my love for You and all the people who surround us until it touches the moon and stars.

Simple Souls

How can You possibly love us so much? Why do You love us so much? Have You always loved us? How long ago did You know we were to be?

I have known you since I was a child. Yet, have I told You enough how much I have loved you? Probably not. For that I am sorry. What simple souls we sometimes are!

Do you realize how wonderful You are? I do.

Mine is just to listen. You will do the rest, I know.

You gave me all that I am. I am grateful.

How can I be a better person? Please direct me.

When I stray, help me to get back on the path that leads to You. That is the path home. Home is where You will be waiting with open arms. I can hardly wait.

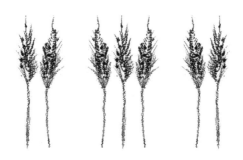

Glory to God

God surrounds us.
   God is everywhere.
   God is listening.
   God is trustworthy.
   God is lovable.
   God is the Father.
   God's son is Jesus Christ.

The Holy Spirit rounds out the Trinity:
   Father, Son, and Holy Spirit.
   Glory be to God in the Trinity.
   Glory to God.

September 11, 2001

Our world turned upside down today. Things will never be the same. I am sorry. You must be horrified. We turn to You for everything. Now, we hardly know what to say. We are silenced by the tragedy. You know our hearts. Please hear them.

Whatever makes some hate? Why do people in far-off lands see others as evil? Is their thinking twisted because we have wounded them in some way? Will there ever be a time when we will all love one another? Will You keep trying to show us how?

Ugliness looms around us. Talk of war and all it includes gets louder. Will striking back solve our problems? Only You know the way. I am sad at the complexity of all that permeates our airways. None of the news includes You. Yet, some speak in Your name. However do we misunderstand what You are truly about? I care. I need to help.

What can I do to make things better? People are collecting money. Cities are coming together to purchase fire trucks, police cars and ambulances. Search dogs sort through the rubble. I watch stunned and helpless.

What can I do to help? My fragile body can't help physically. You see it all in motion from above. Center my thoughts. Put my innocent prayers where they are needed most. I will pray each day that:

people will learn a new kind of love for one another.

hatred will stop.

we will all see You in one another.

our leaders will find a way to heal the hurt we have caused one another.

our world will come together.

we will learn to respect the lives of one another.

each of us will yearn for the happiness of others.

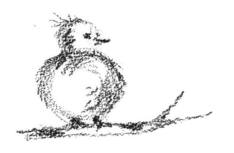

For the Asking

I watched the round, robust, red robin splash its feathered body in the birdbath today. He delighted in the joyful experience You provided for him. When I am able to shower again, I will smile and splash and give thanks for the warm water You have provided for me. As the water runs down my body, I will pray that it will rinse away any wrong I have done. Help me to remember the robin's smile of delightful thanks. When I step from the shower, let me fly to a high branch and chirp the good news to the world. You are available to us for the asking.

Quite Simply

God loves us as babies.
God loves us as children.
God loves us as adolescents.
God loves us as young adults.
God loves us in midlife.
God loves us as we grow old.

God loves us when we are needy.
God loves us when we are anxious.
God loves us when we are sad.
God loves us when we are depressed.
God loves us when we are angry.
God loves us when we are unhappy.

God loves us when we hurt.
God loves us when we are in pain.
God loves us when we are frightened.
God loves us when we are ill.
God loves us when we are uncomfortable.
God loves us when we are very sick.

God loves us even when we are not able to
give Him any attention.

Quite simply, God loves us.

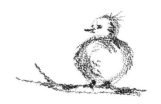

Tiny Am I

- a speck
- a spot
- a semicolon
- a colon
- a flea
- a gnat
- a mosquito
- a period
- a freckle
- a sliver
- a slap
- a pinch
- a pull
- a push
- a tangle
- a knot
- a thread
- a whisker

They all exist with me, and You know us all as tiny as we are. How can that be? You gave us meaning. You love us because we are Your own. Tiny as we are.

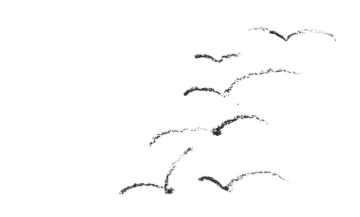

Sweet Spot

Today, I heard the term *sweet spot* for the first time. Sweet spot, I like the sound of it. It stayed with me. I tossed it around in my head. I repeated it several times. Sweet spots? Candy? Cookies? M & M's®? Gumdrops? Jellybeans? No, it is a term used by golf club manufacturers. The sweet spot on a golf club is a spot that makes the golf ball do wonderful things as it flies from the club into the sky.

As I toyed with the idea of a sweet spot, I realized my own sweet spot is in my heart. It is that spot where You always are. It is that spot in me where I harbor Your own sweet self. It is from that "sweet spot" that You make my spirit fly high into the sky reaching for Your goodness and love.

In Love With Life

You gave us early morning. We awake with You by our side. You greet us as we awake.

You help us prepare for our day. We wash and we shower. We get clean. The water You gave us runs freely over our warm skin.

Breakfast is a time for You to prepare us to spend the early day among Your creations. The food of morning nourishes our bodies as thoughts of You nourish our souls.

You accompany us as we start our day: up, down, in, out, speaking, listening, organizing, creating, learning, laboring. Our bodies move in rhythm with our world.

You carry us home again to rest. We repair our tired bodies knowing that You spent the day with us. We nestle in.

There Are Times

There are times I miss who I was.
There are times I miss myself.

There are times when I long for yesterday.
There are times when I yearn for my
   childhood innocence.

There are times when I wish to be
   without pain and worry.
Most of these times are behind me,
   thank heavens.

For now, most of the time is better, because
   most of the time You are near and close.
Being full of You most of the time
   feels good and right.

Thank You for having time for me.
You make me happy, all of the time.

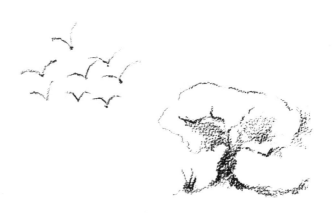

Let Us Not Live in Vain

What would life be like without prayer? What would morning be without Your radiant presence? What would fill the silence of the early hours of awakening? What would the preparations for the day include if there were no joys of Your being with us? High noon without You would be low. Wouldn't afternoons be dreadful without You in our midst?

A world without You at our side is no world at all. It's all so simple. You are our everything. Only with You is there meaning to it all. Glory to God in the highest and peace on earth to the fragile, the sick, the suffering, and the poor souls who do not know Your glory.

Whatever would life be like without You to accept our prayers? Our lives would be in vain. Holy God, receive our prayers. Let us not live in vain.

The Magic of Suffering

There is proof of the magic of my suffering. You gave me this cross to bear that I might be strong in giving to others.

Through this illness, I see the love of others. Through this illness, I feel strong in Your love. Through this illness I get strength

to be honest.

to show my weakness.

to put You first.

to openly talk about Your goodness.

to brighten the lives of others.

to want to learn more.

to be forgiving.

to see good in the smallest of gifts.

And finally, I get strength to laugh at this fragile life with the knowledge and hope of someday living a life in Your presence.

♡ *The prayer of the humble pierces the clouds; it will not rest until it reaches its goal.*

Sirach 35:21

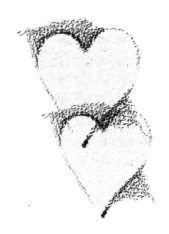

You Love Me as I Am

My hair is gray.
   My forehead is furrowed.
   My eyelids sag.
   My skin is wrinkled.
   My brows are bushy.
   My ear lobes droop.
   My shoulders are humped.
   My chest is caved in.
   My bust no longer tolerates gravity.
   My waist is thick.
   My pelvis is fragile.
   My derriere is gone.
   My legs are fleshless.
   My knees are knobby.
   My ankles are thick.
   My once long, slender feet are full.
   My skin is dry.
   My arms are spotted.

My nails are common.
My wrists are tiny.
My elbows are bony.
My heart is a transplanted heart from some
    dear sweet soul.

I am different from what I was.
Thank You for loving me in spite of the
frailties. They are who I am.

♡ *Gray hair is a crown of glory; it is gained by living a
righteous life.*

Proverbs 16:31

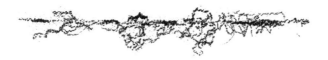

This I Know

Knowing You removes the wondering.
  In You, I know for sure.
  I will hear Your voice.

Tomorrow will come.
  Tomorrow will be a better day.
  I will be healed by Your healing grace.

I will be whole again.
  I will be able to sit by Your side,
  pain free, and filled with the love
  you have promised me.

All this I know for sure.

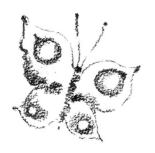

Great Wealth

I am not rich. I am wealthy. There is a big difference. Rich is having things; wealth is knowing love, kindness, peace, joy, tenderness, honesty. You have given me great wealth.

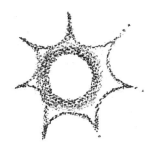

How Was Your Day?

How was Your day today, O Lord? Some of us disappointed You. I pray that I am doing Your will. Lead, that I may go in the direction where I can help You. Teach me how to be more like You. While I have not seen Your face, I know Your hands. They have held me tightly. Let me bring comfort to others with my touch. Let me lighten Your day.

♡ *May God be gracious to us and bless us and make His face to shine upon us.*

Psalm 67:1

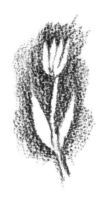

Help Me To Laugh Again

I pray for the gift of laughter. After these years of illness, laughter seems to have quietly slipped away. Make me a lighter soul. Help me to see the bright side of everything.

♡ *The thief comes only to steal, and kill and destroy. I came that they might have life, and have it abundantly.*

John 10:18

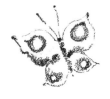

Good-Bye for Now

Shortly, I must say good-bye to a dear friend. He is a twenty-year-old Boston College student. The two of You know one another. He speaks highly of You. The thought of him leaving us for a four-month stay in England is difficult. He is a young man on his own. Letting go is hard. He needs to stretch his wings. His life is his to live.

How ever do You handle letting us go? You gave each of us a free will. On our own, we stumble and fall. You are always there when we call. You give us the freedom to stretch our wings. However do You stand it?

You love us more than we know, yet You do not force us to know and to love You. We come to You freely.

When my Boston College buddy arrives in England,

please be with him. Just as You greet me each day, stand by him. He is young; You are wise. Speak softly to him. When difficulties arise, show him the way. He will not be alone in a foreign land, for You are at his side. Love and protect him as he grows into the man he is sure to be.

You taught us how to say good-bye. Life is full of good-byes. As we get closer to our heavenly destination, the good-byes of this world will change. Those who have gone before will greet us, and there will be no more good-byes.

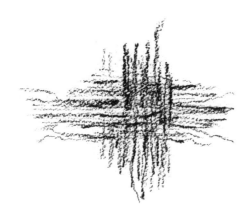

There Are No Bad Times

You protect us by always being at our side.
You protect us by always trusting
   what we have to say.

You give us a way to see the truth.
You whisper which direction we should go
   when we get lost.

You shield us from a difficult world.
You are always our friend.

Your soften our hearts.
You have promised us eternity.

Thank You, Lord.

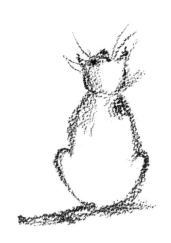

Your Creation

The cat curls round in his favorite basket. His eyes etch two tight lines on his furry face. As he sleeps, his whiskers wiggle and twitch. His fuzzy ears poke above the basket just enough to display their symmetrical perfection.

You gave him to me that I would know of Your creative wonders. In his elegance, he delights in a ray of sunshine. He needs little to appreciate Your goodness.

Help me to be more like him. Teach me his simple, sure ways. Make me content, as he is content. He is here that I might examine his perfection.

His simplicity startles me most. He gracefully moves through his day as smoothly as the sun moves through the sky. You show me the way, in the most remarkable of situations. Fill me with his ease of grace. I will follow that ray of sunshine. I will work to develop simple, sure ways. I will follow his simplicity. I will follow his silence.

♡ *Blessed be the Lord, for He has heard the sound of my pleading, the Lord is my strength and my shield; in Him my heart trusts; so I am helped and my heart exults, and with my song I give thanks to Him.*

Psalm 27:6–7

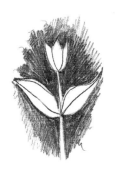

Conclusion

When Jerry and I attend a party or go with friends to dinner, or attend church, I have a difficult time leaving. I find a terrible need to touch each person no matter the size of the group. I desire to look into the eyes of each. I hate saying good-bye.

Jerry always teases me. When we finally get to our car, he always remarks that he thought I'd never get my good-byes finished. I have this terrible need to make sure they know that I love them and that they see You in me.

Jerry has learned to start an hour early to prepare for our departure. I seem always to have just one more hopeful, caring part of myself to leave behind.

Today, I have felt that same feeling. It's time for *For the*

Asking: A Joyful Journey to Peace to come to an end. Yet, I want to go on.

I loved sharing my own prayers and stories with you. I need you to know that illness brings with it a kind of prayer that only those who have known real pain know. I have this desire to share, to give, to encourage, to help you as you walk the same journey I have made.

When I began this little venture, I was timid. I was in terrible pain. I was confused. Today I have those days behind me. Along with them has gone the pain. I am no longer timid about telling people about the gifts of God. I am not confused about the business of illness.

My need to help others find hope during some of the worst of times has led me to today. The prayer of the ill, the injured, the wounded, and the dying are the prayers of life. It has taken me years to come to where I am. And while I have taken but small steps, I have moved forward. I can feel the peace in my spiritual growth.

Take joy in who you are. You are never far from the grandest friend you have. God is waiting to hear you say hello as I now say my good-bye.

♡ *Leave in good time and do not be the last; go home quickly and do not linger.*

Sirach 32:11

Happy are those who hear You.

There is no end to Your greatness!

I will listen and I will follow.

So be it.

Farewell for now, my friends,
Kathleen